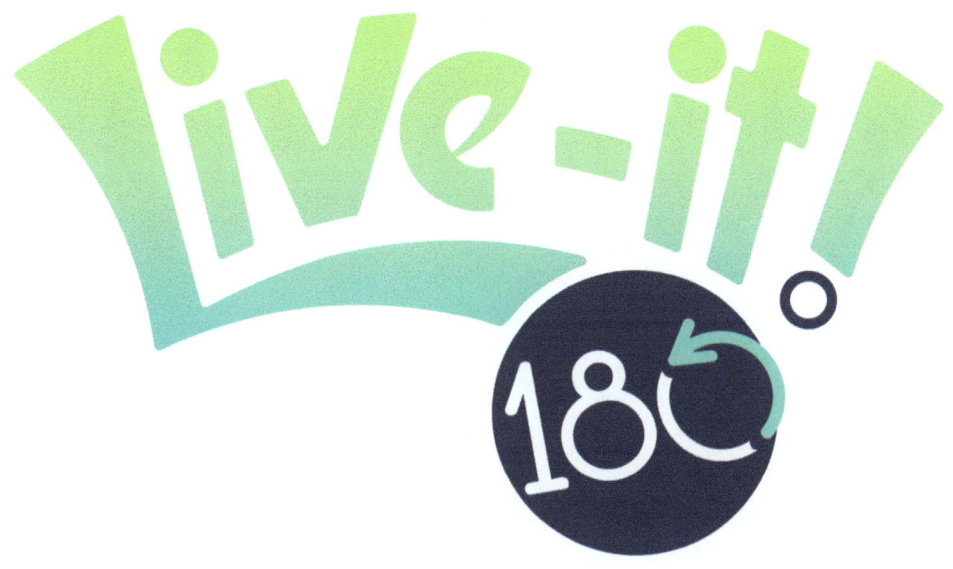

Your body's intelligent design for
losing weight, *living fit*, and *enjoying life!*

PETER H. JENNINGS

Copyright © Live-it! 180°
All rights reserved, including the right to reproduce this book or portions thereof in any form whatsoever.

Live-it! 180°
111 Charles St.
Manchester, NH 03101

Author: Peter Jennings
Editor: Safie Maken Finlay
Graphic Designer: Kaylee Kelso

Credits:
Jennings Photos and Food Portion Photos
Stacey Brobst Photographer

Cover photo:
Istock.com

All other photos:
Unsplash.com
BigStock.com

Library and Archives
Jennings, Peter H., 2019-
      Live-it! 180° : Your body's intelligent design for losing weight, living fit, and enjoying life! / Peter H. Jennings

ISBN 9780578523194

      1. Health and hygiene. 2. Lifestyle. 3. Weight loss. 4. Reducing diets.

IMPORTANT
The information in this book reflects the author's experience and opinions. It is NOT intended to replace medical advice.

The material in this book is not meant to diagnose, treat, or cure any medical condition. The material is not intended to replace the advice of your physician. Before beginning, this or any nutritional or exercise regimen, consult your physician.

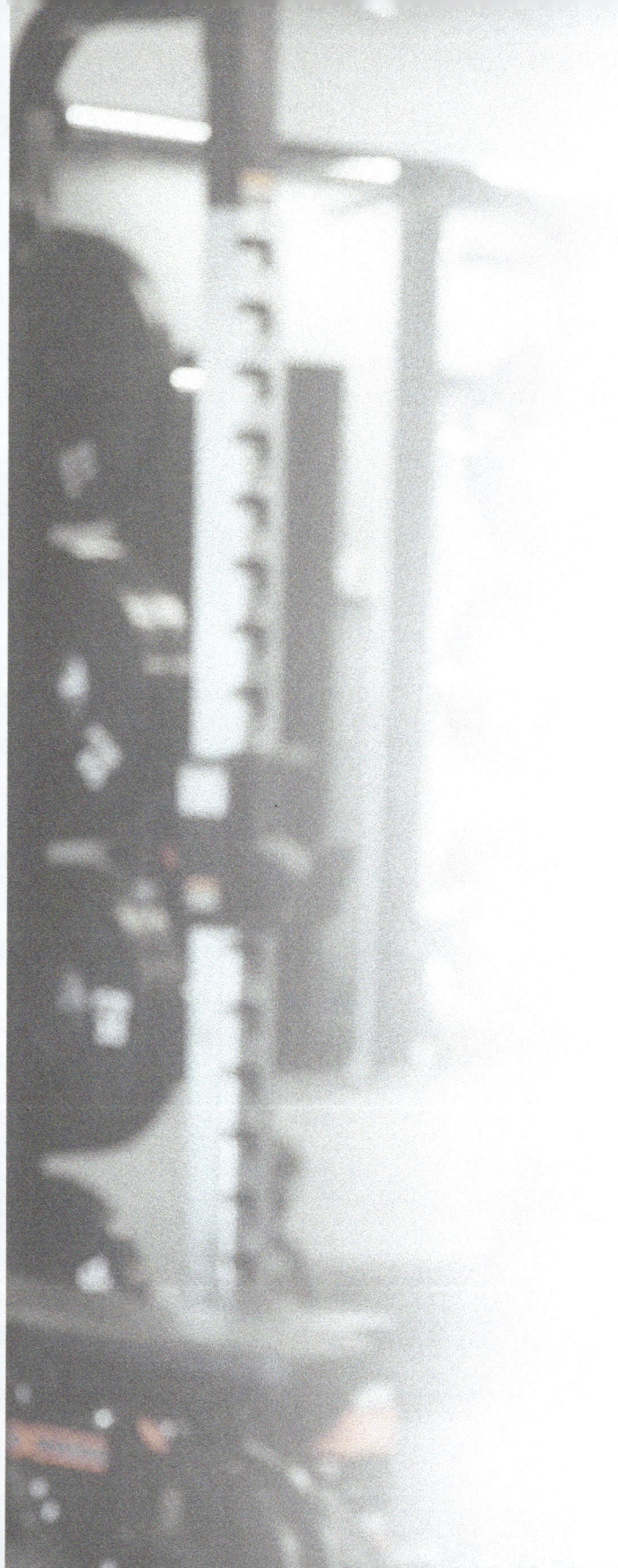

DEDICATION

First I'd like to thank God the Father and my Lord Jesus Christ for making me, designing me, and enabling me to take on this endeavor. I have been abundantly blessed with my gifts, talents, intelligence, faith, a beautiful wife, awesome kids, businesses, and friendships. To much has been given, much is expected.

In writing this book, countless hours of my time reading and researching, testing each diet, lifestyle, and healthy concepts, and my family signing up for for the challenge of taking on this endeavor with me as my support and guinea pigs, I'm forever thankful and indebted to them.

I dedicate this book to the love of my life, the most beautiful woman on the planet, my Proverbs 31 girl, my wife for life, Nadia, and to the best kids a father could ever ask for, Joshua, Nakahla, Emma, Lydia, and Vaughn. My family is my life and the reason I decided to take this journey and write Live-It! 180°. They are my inspiration that caused me to want to "live-it" everyday. I am gratefully and eternally thankful for everyone of you. I Love and adore you all.

There are several individuals, of which I could write a whole separate book on, who have inspired me and listened to me rant about about all the stuff I discovered. I dedicate this book to them also, my sister Susan (who I couldn't live without), my friends (Adam, Peter, Phil, Neil, Kyle) and also Dr.

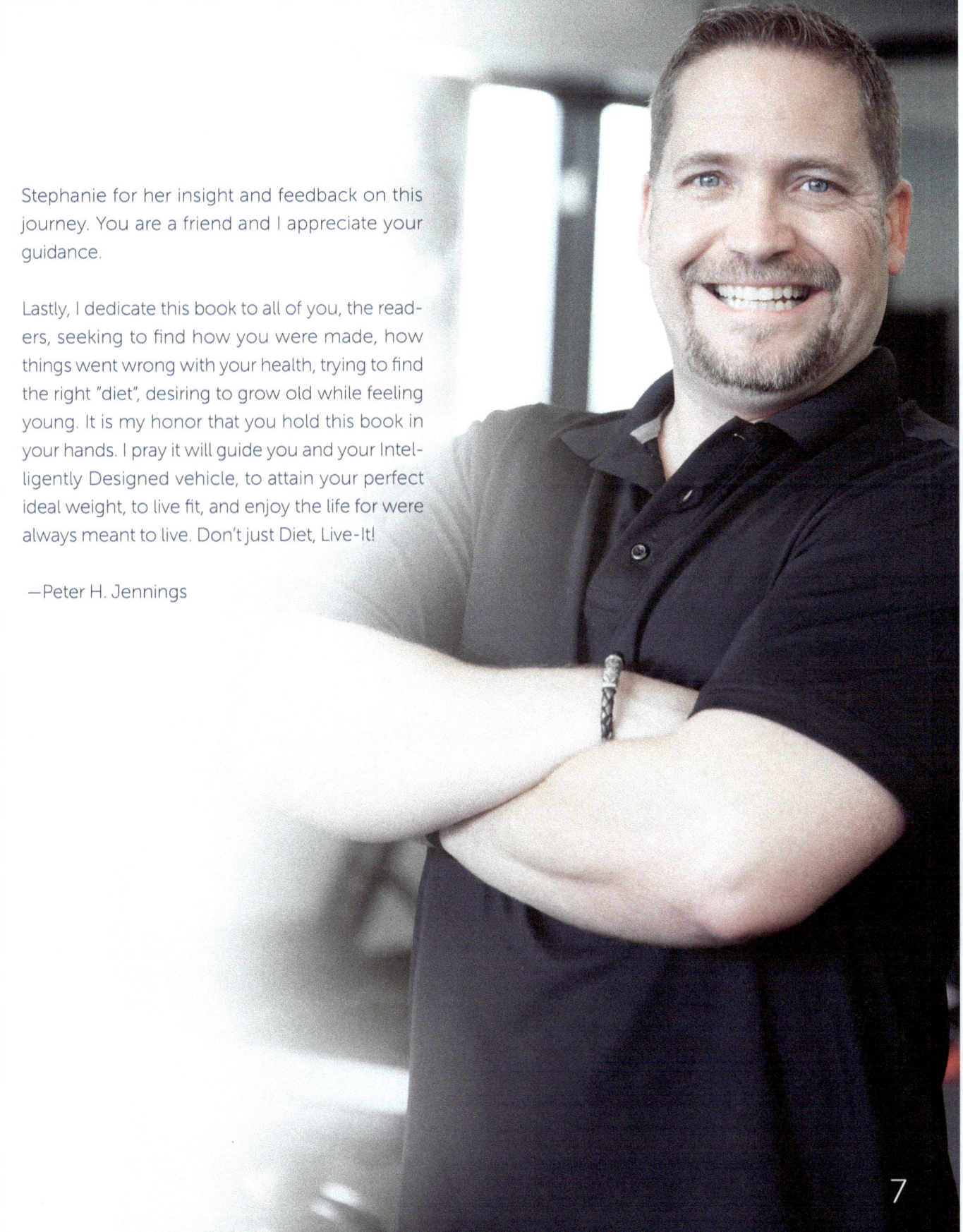

Stephanie for her insight and feedback on this journey. You are a friend and I appreciate your guidance.

Lastly, I dedicate this book to all of you, the readers, seeking to find how you were made, how things went wrong with your health, trying to find the right "diet", desiring to grow old while feeling young. It is my honor that you hold this book in your hands. I pray it will guide you and your Intelligently Designed vehicle, to attain your perfect ideal weight, to live fit, and enjoy the life for were always meant to live. Don't just Diet, Live-It!

—Peter H. Jennings

CONTENTS

	Foreward	10
Chapter 1	THE WAKE-UP CALL	13
	It's All About the Choices	15
	What Works?	24
	Redefining the Word "Diet"	26
Chapter 2	MY REQUEST TO YOU	33
	Three Big Life Lessons	34
Chapter 3	INTELLIGENT DESIGN	37
	You Are Not an Accident	39
	Are You Sabotaging the Intelligently Designed Autopilot/Conductor?	44
Chapter 4	A BRIEF OVERVIEW OF LIVE-IT! 180°	47
	Tapping into Your Body's Ability to Heal Itself	49
	The Five Critical Habits	51
	Accountability	54
	The LIVE-IT! 180° House Plan	57
Chapter 5	RECHARGE	59
	What Happens When you Mess Up Your Battery?	63
	Challenge the Status Quo	66
	The Basics: What You Need to Know about Your Sleep Pattern	68
	GOOD, BETTER, **BEST**: Personalize LIVE-IT! 180°	71
Chapter 6	FUEL	75
	What Big Food Doesn't Want You to Know	77
	What to Eat, How Much to Eat, When to Eat	87
	Four Daily Supplements	99
	GOOD, BETTER, **BEST**: Personalize LIVE-IT! 180°	103

Chapter 7	DRIVE	111
	This Can Be an Emotional Issue!	112
	Why This Is So Important: The Sludge Factor	113
	The Aging Myth	121
	The Advantages of Movement	123
	GOOD, BETTER, **BEST**:	
	Personalize LIVE-IT! 180°	128
Chapter 8	CONNECT	133
	Close up on the Okinawa Culture	140
	Yet Another Benefit of Connecting	141
	GOOD, BETTER, **BEST**:	
	Personalize LIVE-IT! 180°	145
Chapter 9	REPAIR	151
	Eustress and Distress, Revisited	154
	Starting Simple	152
	GOOD, BETTER, **BEST**:	
	Personalize LIVE-IT! 180°	159
Chapter 10	GETTING STARTED WITH THE	
	LIVE-IT! 180° SYSTEM	165
	Why This Is Different	167
	Three Guidelines	167
Epilogue		189
Appendix	CLOSE-UP ON YOUR KITCHEN MAKEOVER	193
	Putting Together Your Weekly Grocery List	205

FOREWORD

According to the World Health Organization, over 70% of deaths in the year 2020 will be due to chronic diseases like heart disease, obesity, and diabetes. The figure will be even higher in developed nations like the United States... and it's important to note that we can just as easily call these chronic diseases "diseases of lifestyle." They are rooted in the choices we make about the way we live.

(Source: http://www.who.int/nutrition/topics/2_background/en/)

This troubling trend connects to a related, largely unexamined, and all-too-inevitable truth: The modern American way of life -- the default patterns by which most of us shop, eat, sleep, move, and interact with each other -- is fundamentally unhealthy.

We need to understand this. The familiar American lifestyle -- sedentary, convenient, increasingly isolated, and all too often driven by the commercial interests of large industries -- lowers the quality of our lives and leads us to needlessly early deaths. That is the reality of life in the USA in the early twenty-first century.

For a variety of reasons, most Americans are unaware, confused, or blissfully ignorant about what it means to live a truly healthy lifestyle. Too many of us imagine that living a healthy lifestyle means making a few superficial changes in the way we live, like following the latest popular "diet plan." Making a few temporary changes in the foods we eat isn't enough... but most of us won't realize that until it's too late.

Dorland's Medical Dictionary defines health as "a condition of optimum physical, social, mental and spiritual well-being – not merely the absence of disease or infirmities." It takes more than clean eating to be healthy. It takes a series of fundamental changes in the choices you make in your physical, social, mental, and spiritual life.

The LIVE-IT! 180° program will make it easier for you to make those choices. This isn't a fad diet or exercise program. It is a comprehensive, yet accessible beginner's guide that will move you toward total well-being in a holistic way. It will not ask you to change everything overnight, but neither will it pretend there are short-cuts or quick fixes on the way to a longer, happier, healthy life. This book gives you the knowledge, the action steps, and (most important of all) the reasons to make lifestyle changes that are sustainable.

Most diet and fitness programs stop at just that, exercise and/or fitness. They don't address the underlying issues that cause poor eating habits and lack of motivation to exercise. In effect, most programs become a treatment for the symptom of overweight, not a makeover for your lifestyle. If stress, human connections, sleep, and mindset are not addressed, the changes become only a temporary fix, not a long-term solution.

In this unique program, all areas of health are seen as what they are: interconnected. If one aspect is left unaddressed, the other parts will suffer. By addressing all aspects of a healthy lifestyle, in a system that is easy to understand and implement, LIVE-IT 180 allows you to make sustainable changes that will last. It gives you practical strategies for making better choices that will help you to create your best self.

So, find a partner ... and get started. No prior experience is necessary. Right now, a healthier, happier, more abundant life -- your ideal life, the life you were meant to live -- is waiting for you to LIVE-IT!

—Dr. Stephanie Mills,
Chiropractor

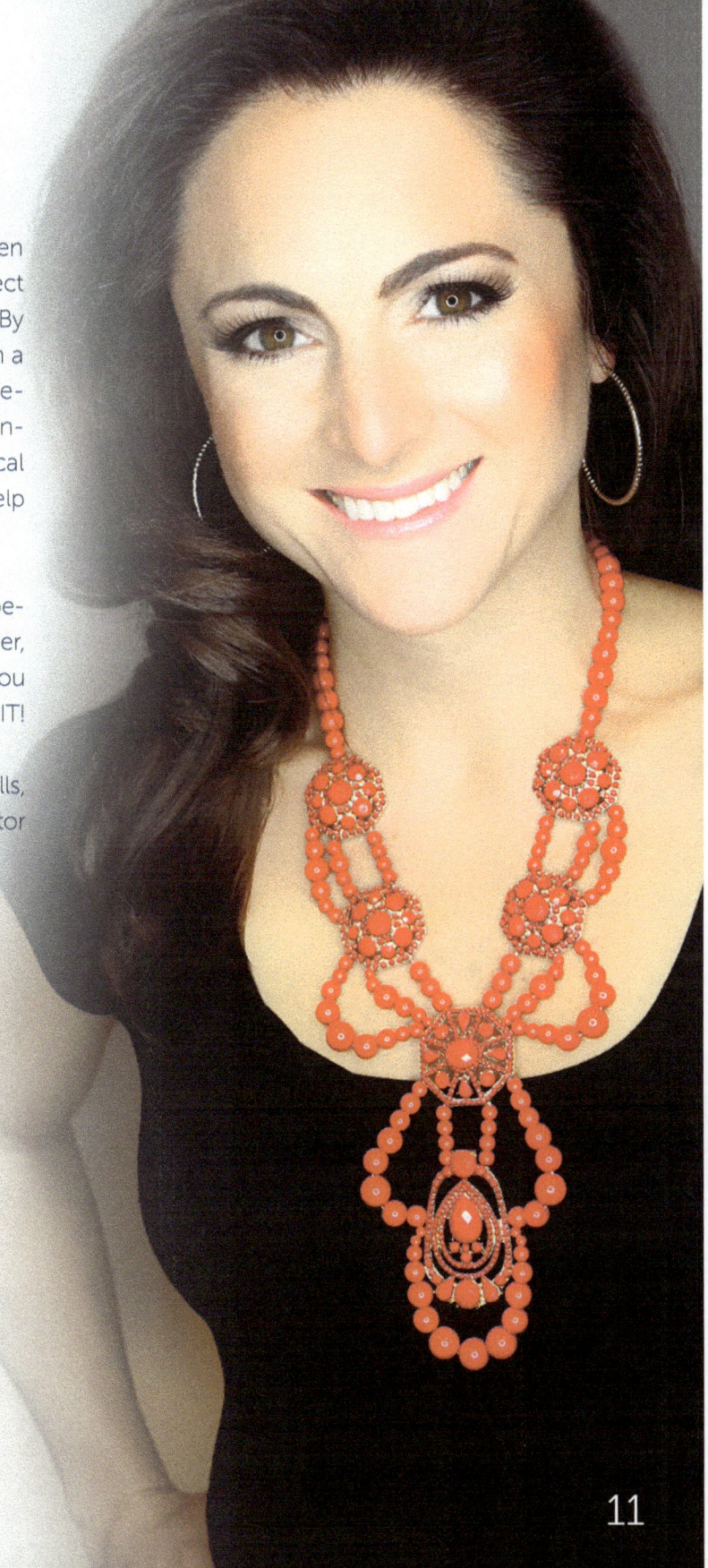

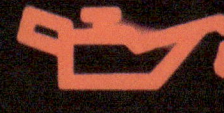

THE WAKE-UP CALL

The big problem was that he was overweight. And he wasn't doing anything to fix that problem.

He was forty years old, five feet eight inches tall, and he tipped the scales at 215 pounds. (The ideal weight for a man of his height and muscle structure is around 180.) He was the CEO of a national firm. He had a couple of homes. He took regular vacations. His wife and kids were healthy and loved him dearly. He was active in his church. He told everyone how happy he was, and he tried, without much success, to convince himself that this was true. He thought he was leading a successful life because he was financially successful. And he assumed that meant he must be happy. But he was wrong. He was desperately unhappy, and deep down he knew that the main reason he was unhappy was that he was overweight. But he didn't have time to try to turn that situation around. He was too busy.

He knew the extra weight he was carrying around had all kinds of negative effects on his life. He was constantly tired and depressed. He usually felt like he had no energy. He hadn't slept well in months. His blood work was a disaster. He had constant aches and pains, strange kidney issues, tightness in his chest, a failing gallbladder, and high blood pressure. Thick layers of fat pushed down, in, and onto all his organ systems. This meant he often felt out of sorts and uncomfortable, which was one of the big reasons he had difficulty sleeping. He looked lousy in a bathing suit, and although he kept trying to tell himself how much he loved his work and how devoted he was to his family, deep inside, a little voice he tried to pretend he couldn't hear gave him this message:

Hey – you're making a big mistake. You need to take better care of yourself. You need to lose some weight.

That little voice, which he had successfully ignored for over a decade, turned out to be absolutely right. I can say that because the guy in question happened to be very, very close to me.

In fact, he *was* me!

A CONVERSATION WITH THE MIRROR

During this difficult period of my life, I would sometimes look at my overweight self in the mirror, and not liking what I saw, silently ask my reflection, *How did you get to this point?*

After all, for years I had been leading a healthy, happy lifestyle and helping others to do the same. I had worked hard – very hard – and made my company a success. I made good money. I had a caring, beautiful, supportive wife, great kids (largely because I was totally committed to them and eager to provide for them), and a career other people envied. I shuttled the kids around – between school and home and lessons and home and soccer games and home – and basically lived the American dream.

Yet I was also living the American nightmare.

I got little or no exercise. I hurtled from meeting to meeting in my car, ate fast food on the run, and worked way too many twelve- and fourteen-hour days. My stress levels were through the roof. My life was chaotic and stressful and unbalanced, but I hid that fact from everyone I loved. When people asked how I was doing, I said things were great ... but deep down, part of me knew darn well from the look of my reflection in the mirror that things weren't great at all.

I needed to lose weight, and I had been ignoring that reality for years. Now I was in trouble, and I could sense that the trouble was getting worse. I tried to tune out the voice that kept telling me there was a problem and listen exclusively to the voice that said things were going great. I tried to tune out the headaches, the chest pains, the abdominal pains, the insomnia.

Then came my wake-up call.

IT'S ALL ABOUT THE CHOICES

Mother Nature is relentless. If she notices you making stupid choices, she will call you and continue calling you, patiently waiting for you to pick up the line. She will give you all kinds of signals designed to tell you that it's time to take a time-out and start changing your life ... by making better choices. She will send you warning notices

> "Then came my wake-up call."

marked URGENT ... and like the warning lights on your car's dashboard, if you ignore them, things will begin to break down.

If you keep staring into the mirror and doing nothing about what you see ... if you *continue* to make stupid choices ... Mother Nature will start dropping more obvious, more impossible-to-ignore hints. She'll make it increasingly difficult for you to ignore her message: that it's time for you to stop choosing what's hurting you and start choosing what's good for you, what's healthy, what's right, what's *designed* for you. Our bodies are designed to protect us, even from ourselves. Eventually, Mother Nature will flash *lots* of red lights on your body's dashboard.

And you know what? If you ignore those flashing red lights for long enough, Mother Nature has no problem going to the next level. She will shut you down.

In my case, I ignored the lights on the dashboard for a very long time, and Mother Nature went to the next level. In 2012, at 5:30 on a bitterly cold winter morning, she sent me into agony.

The wind was howling outside, loud enough to shatter the thin, brittle film of sleep in which I'd been trying, and failing, to seek refuge from my own body. I knew from the previous night's news

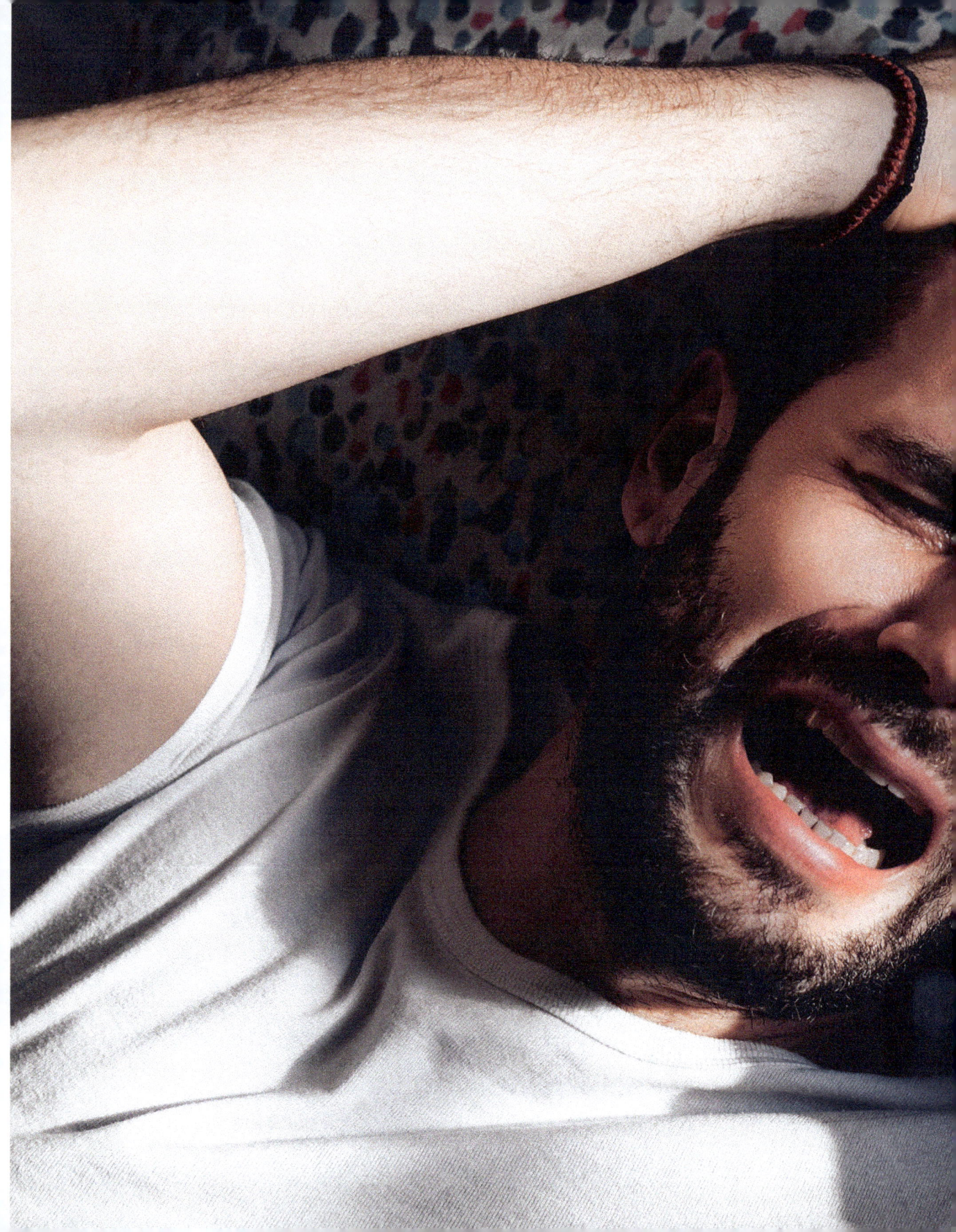

reports that the windchill outside was likely to be well south of fifteen degrees below zero, and I could hear trees coming down. Our power had flickered on and off all through the night, and when I forced the caked lids of my eyes open and glanced out my window, I saw that the panes were rimmed with thick layers of frost. A big storm had indeed blown in and left in its wake a maze of distressed tree limbs, either hanging low with ice or tangled and dismembered, blocking the pathways outside.

Then something fiery stabbed me from inside.

I hadn't been sleeping well for weeks (remember what I said a little earlier about warning lights on the dashboard?), and this past evening had been particularly unbearable. My pain and discomfort had grown so intense that it was now not only impossible to pretend I was getting the rest I needed, it was impossible to breathe. I felt like someone was jabbing me in my back, stomach, and groin with a hot poker. It was as if fiery shards of glass were being forced through my veins.

What was going on?

I rolled out of bed and slumped onto the floor, crouching on my hands and knees with tears in my eyes. I gasped out to my wife, Nadine, "Help me. Call the ambulance!" I remained in a fetal position, rocking back and forth, breathing my way through each new wave of sharp, nearly overwhelming pain as she made the call.

"What was going on? I wondered if I was dying."

I wondered if I was dying.

I lay there on the floor, moaning and rocking and weeping, until the ambulance arrived. It took a while. (They had to clear away some of those fallen tree limbs to get to our house.)

When the paramedics made their way to my room, they put me on a stretcher, carted me out of the house and into that freezing air, and loaded me into the back of the vehicle. My wife had to stay behind with the kids. (She told me later that when she looked at me being loaded into the ambulance, she thought it might be the last time she saw me.) Once I was strapped in, the assessment began. There was a barrage of questions from one of the paramedics, most of which I didn't even understand, and a barrage of poking from another paramedic, most of it painful.

Just about every inch of my body hurt now. I tried my best to answer the questions I could make sense of, but no matter what I said, the pain kept stabbing me from inside. I saw that I was being hooked up to some kind of machine they had inside the ambulance, or maybe a complex series of machines. I remember that there were wires everywhere I looked.

I remember everything hurting.

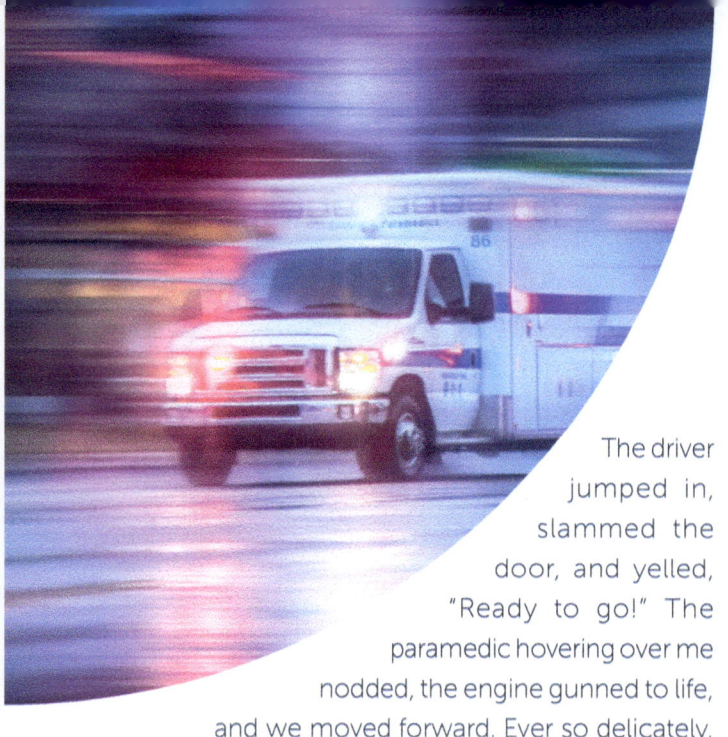

The driver jumped in, slammed the door, and yelled, "Ready to go!" The paramedic hovering over me nodded, the engine gunned to life, and we moved forward. Ever so delicately, the driver navigated his way down our perilous, icy driveway. The exit to the main road had never felt so agonizing.

The trip to the emergency room seemed to take forever, because the ice on the road was so treacherous, and the driver, to his credit, didn't want to end up in a ditch. As we pressed ahead, the waves of pain convulsing my body grew more intense, and my breathing grew shorter and more labored.

Was this it? Was I going to die before we even made it to the emergency room?

I decided to stop focusing on that fear and to start focusing my mental capacity on a slightly less terrifying question: What in the world was going wrong with my body?

WHAT WAS HAPPENING TO ME?

All I could think of was that there was a war raging inside me, a war that was moving very quickly indeed and that my body was losing. I remember thinking that the only people who could figure out what was going on were the doctors waiting for me at the emergency room. They would figure it out. They would help me.

We finally arrived at the hospital. After I was unwired from whatever machinery the paramedics had been using to monitor me, I was wheeled on my mobile stretcher into the emergency room, where the barrage of questions continued. All my gasped-out answers seemed to miss the mark. The poking also continued, only now I was being poked with even greater vigor by a larger number of people with more strange tools at their disposal. I remember being stabbed with hypodermic needles. I also remember feeling like I wanted to give up on life, something I had never felt before.

Fortunately, one of those hypodermic needles carried a large dose of painkiller, and the pain began to subside. I began to feel that help had finally arrived.

Thank God for painkillers.

I could draw this story out — sharing all the fascinating, difficult, disgusting things that happened to me at the hospital that day — but this chapter is not about the details of that day. It is about my personal wake-up call. This came when the doctors finally figured out what was happening to me. They discovered that I had multiple kidney stones.

> **KIDNEY STONES: What does that mean?**
>
> Kidney stones are rock-hard deposits of minerals and salts that form inside your kidneys. This typically happens when the urine becomes highly concentrated in a way that allows minerals and salts to crystallize and stick together. Basically, what happens is that too many toxins accumulate for your body to break down, producing tiny pebbles that assault your kidney, bladder, and urinary tract as they pass through … creating waves of exquisite pain that get steadily worse. The pain assaults your back, side, abdomen, groin, and/or genitals. Those who have passed a single kidney stone often describe the ordeal as, "the worst pain I've ever felt." I had multiple stones to pass. And yes, it was the worst pain I've ever experienced.

My condition was more agonizing than words I type out on a computer screen could ever convey. All I can tell you is that I hope and pray that nothing even remotely similar to my wake-up call ever happens in your life. (Eventually, Nadine and I realized we had to do a whole lot more than hope if we wanted to make sure that what happened to me didn't happen to other people. But I'm getting ahead of myself.)

WHOSE PROBLEM WAS THIS?

In the immediate aftermath of my trip to the emergency room, I still didn't recognize that what had happened to me was due to my own choices. That's how powerful the human denial instinct can be. I didn't connect the kidney stones to all the extra pounds I was carting around every day. Even when I was confronted directly with the reality of my situation, I did what a lot of people who suddenly find themselves very, very sick tend to do: I put the onus for fixing the problem on the medical establishment.

After passing those stones (an experience I would not wish on my worst enemy) and after several weeks of seemingly pointless tests and exams, I remember getting a bit impatient. At one point, I said to my doctor, "Listen. I've got a company to run. Am I over the hump?"

The look the doctor gave me in response indicated anything but YES. I decided to rephrase the question. "What I mean to say is, Now what? Where do I go from here?"

He gave me another odd look, sadder this time, and said, "Peter, come with me. I want to show you something."

I shrugged my shoulders and said, "Sure," uncertain where this was leading. When was the doctor going to let me get back to work? Wasn't that what this was all about?

I followed him into a dimly lit examination room. There, after closing the door, he pointed toward a display on the wall. It was the strangest thing I had ever seen in my entire life. The wall was lined with dozens and dozens of small, capped glass tubes filled with what looked like urine.

"We call this the Wall of Shame," my doctor said. "Every single one of these glass tubes is filled with the pee of some stressed-out guy who didn't take care of himself and who got himself into just the kind of agony that you experienced a while back. Each of these tubes is from someone in a high-stress position, someone like you, who saw himself headed for the edge of a cliff and kept right on flooring the accelerator. Some high-powered executive. Or firefighter. Or policeman. Now, here's the reason I'm showing you this. The tubes are arranged in order, from best to worst. What I want you to notice is that yours is at the end of the line, right before the last tube. That last tube came from another CEO, by the way. He didn't make it. So, you ask me when you're going back to work, as though that were the problem. I've got news for you. That's not the problem. The problem is this: Your tube is now officially the worst sample we have from a living person. The question you and I need to consider right now is this: Are you going to join your fellow CEO in the Dead Executives Society ... or are you going to start making better choices, lose some weight, and stick around for a while?"

Gulp.

Seeing that he had got my attention, the doctor gestured for me to take a seat. Once I did, he sat down too and looked me straight in the eye.

"Are you with me so far, Peter?"

"Yes."

"Are you sure?"

"Yes."

"Good. Now, I can tell you're a bottom-line kind of guy, which can sometimes make this discussion a little easier. So, I'll get straight to the point. Here's your bottom line. You got lucky this time. But if you don't change your life, starting right now – meaning dropping a significant amount of weight – you can't count on being so lucky next time. From now on, you must start making better choices. Your body is like a car on autopilot, heading toward a cliff. You need to do a 180 degree turn immediately. And by the way, this change depends on you. Not on me. On you."

Okay, Mother Nature. You had got my attention! It was time to lose some weight.

> "You had got my attention! It was time to lose some weight."

THIS SHOULDN'T HAVE HAPPENED

I want to reiterate now what I couldn't accept before that little chat with my doctor: What happened to me was my own responsibility and nobody else's. I was the one who let my weight get out of control. I was the one who made consistently terrible choices about my own health. The choices we make today determine our future. Choose wisely!

The major irony in my situation was that I was probably the last person on earth you would expect to have a major weight problem and multiple kidney stones. I was – and am – a serious fitness guy. I really, really, really should have known better than to let myself go to such a degree. At the time my doctor gave me that little pep talk, I was maybe the best-informed, best-trained, most-credentialed seriously overweight guy in that hospital: a fourth-degree black belt who had studied nutrition, stress management, physiology, neurology, and soft-tissue damage repair in depth. I was knowledgeable in many aspects of health, wellness, and healing. From a very young age, I had trained myself in anatomy and the inner workings of the human body. After graduating from the New Hampshire Institute for Wholistic Health, I became licensed as a therapist and worked for an accomplished New England chiropractor for four years. I subsequently opened the Occipital Coccyx Neuromuscular Massage Therapy Center, where I successfully helped over 320 clients to heal their soft-tissue issues.

The Center was a huge success, helping many people make the journey back to health. We had 80 appointments a week, specializing in soft tissue issues and nutrition consulting. Over 50 different doctors and other practitioners referred their patients to us. Over the course of the year the Center was open, I found that my treatments weren't the only things helping my clients. My specialized massages provided substantial relief from pain or soft tissue damage, but I learned that there was much, much more to the human body, to health and living vibrantly, than stress management and deep tissue work.

Some common ground started to emerge in my clients' success stories. I noticed that along with

the massages, getting enough sleep, good nutrition, exercise, stress management, social relationships, and a commitment to stay on track with all these things appeared to have major benefits. As my practice grew, these truths started to present themselves more and more powerfully.

As I said, I should have known better.

One night a fire broke out at our facility. Although no one was hurt, the blaze burned our building very badly. I should point out that I am a firm believer that in human life, everything has a season. Family, friends, work – all these things go through periods of transition. Nothing lasts forever. When one chapter closes, another one begins. So, when I was presented with the challenge of my building burning down, I did a reassessment and decided, after a good deal of thought, to close the business and make a career change.

I was ready for a new chapter to open in my life. I was about to get married. I wanted more financial security than I had while working at the therapy center. An opportunity had come my way to work for a large national firm selling financial services, life insurance, and mutual funds. I decided to accept the offer. I was ready for a change – in fact, I welcomed it.

I'm compressing a lot in what follows, but the Cliff's Notes version of what happened over the next few years is pretty important, so please stay with me. After jumping into this new career, I worked hard (as you've probably gathered, I'm pretty good at

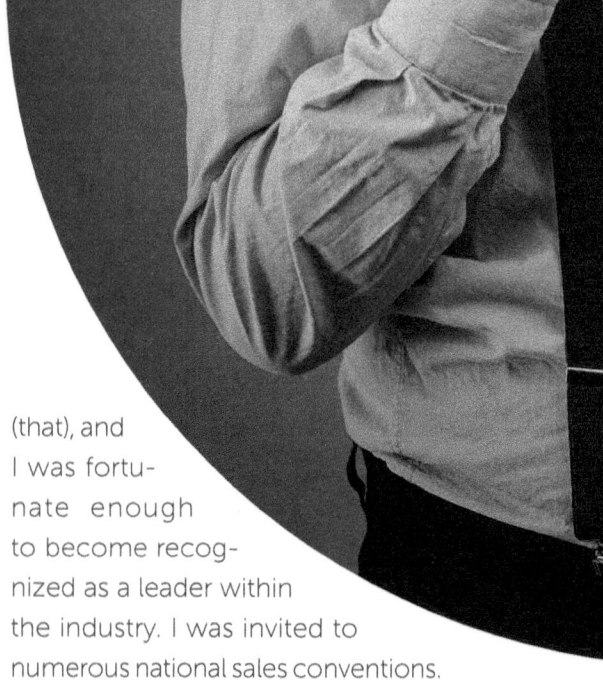

(that), and I was fortunate enough to become recognized as a leader within the industry. I was invited to numerous national sales conventions. I won some sales awards. I did a fair amount of keynote speaking. The upshot was that I began to be able to provide my wife and growing family with the security I had wanted to give them.

Life was good, and I was blessed. After a while, I was recruited to a new, growing firm in the benefit administration industry, where the blessings continued. Before long, I was recognized as one of the top sales agents in the country. This meant more travel, more conventions, more awards, more money, and more speeches. In short, it meant life was going where I wanted it to go. It seemed obvious to me that I had made the right decision to leave the therapy business and pursue a fast-track career in the financial/benefits field, and I suppose from one perspective I had.

But I was overlooking something important: my own health. Although this new chapter of my life had propelled me forward financially, the fast track I was on was causing me to make choices that didn't

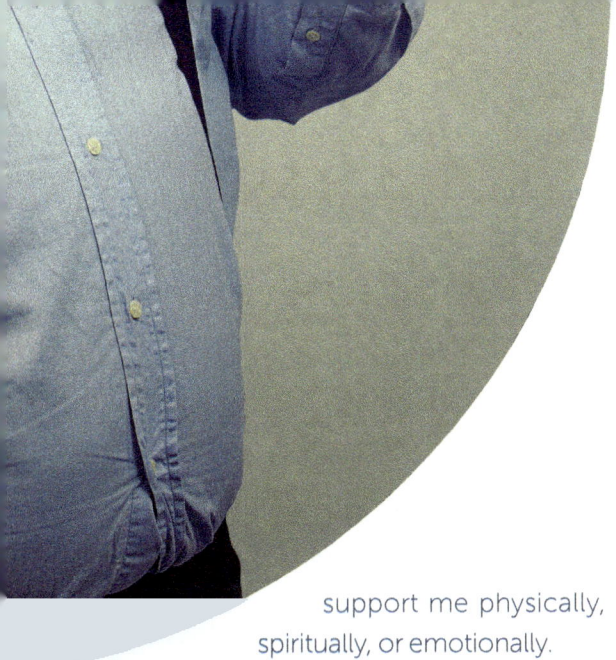

support me physically, spiritually, or emotionally.

I started gaining weight. Lots of weight.

I barely noticed that I had moved away from the habits I once lived by as a "fitness guy" – the habits of staying on track with what my body needed in terms of what I ate, how I slept, the kind of exercise I got, and so on. Although I was focused like a laser beam on financial success, I was setting myself up for disaster on just about every other front that mattered to me and my family.

This impending disaster did not become obvious to me until I got my wake-up call from Mother Nature. In the meantime, I consumed massive amounts of fast food, dehydrated myself, drove a lot, walked very little, and spent way too many long hours on the job.

Let me break down the next phase in the decade of abuse I put my body through. In 2002, after due consideration, I decided to move back into the entrepreneurial world, this time by starting my very own benefit administration business. The firm grew quickly and by 2005, we were a multi-million-dollar company. More good news, right?

Well, that's what I thought at the time. What was not to like about my life? I was now the CEO of a successful, fast-growing company. I was happily married, and I had a great family. I had attained a high level of financial success, and that success was escalating. My wife and I were investing in a range of startups, and those investments were paying off. It all sounded great on paper.

But I was headed for the cliff, with my foot jammed down on the accelerator.

The more "successful" I got, the harder I worked. The more I worked, the worse I slept and the more junk food I ate. The longer my hours at work became, the more isolated and stressed-out I felt and the more weight I gained.

To her eternal credit, Nadine warned me repeatedly about the consequences of the choices I was making. She tried her best to convince me to change course. But I chose not to listen.

There came a point where everything in my life, with the exception of my marriage, was radically out of balance. Why? Because I was ignoring what I had once helped other people to master in their lives. Years of worsening insomnia, bad diet, little or no exercise, cursory social connections outside of my family unit, and endless, thundering tidal waves of negative stress all finally caught up with me that brutally cold winter morning when I got my wake-up call. I was overweight and in deep trouble by that point, and the reason for all that trouble was looking back at me in every mirror I passed.

So, after a decade of sabotaging my own body, I experienced that reality-check moment, the moment when my doctor challenged me to take a close look at my spot on the Wall of Shame and ask myself another tough question:

Am I serious about losing weight?

I decided that I was serious. I resolved to put as much effort and energy into losing the weight I needed to lose as I had into becoming financially successful. I got my mind set on a new goal: I was going to lose the extra pounds and keep them off – period. I knew this was going to be a major undertaking. To make sure I followed through on my weight loss goal, I got myself an accountability partner: my wife. I shared my goal with Nadine. She agreed to help me and support me as I followed through and pursued that goal. And thank God she did, because there were times when the going got pretty rough.

WHAT WORKS?

I became a guinea pig. My body, I decided, was going to be the laboratory. I was going to find out, one way or another, what worked when it came to losing weight and keeping it off. That's what I needed to do, right?

Over the next four years, I tried every popular diet program I could get my hands on. And I do mean every one. You may think I'm kidding. I'm not. If it had mainstream success, if people were saying good things about it, and if it seemed to be delivering good results for real, live people, I wanted to know if it would work for me. I tracked it down, studied it, figured out exactly what the plan wanted me to do, and then implemented the plan to the letter.

I tried the Maker's diet, whose tagline is, "what would Jesus eat?" By the way – that's a very good question, which is worth considering closely! If you think Jesus would have been okay with heavily processed food and lots of chemical additives, which are added to make a company's bottom line look better at the expense of human beings, I have to disagree. Even though I was in line with the diet spiritually and philosophically, it wasn't what I was looking for. It worked for a while ... I got some good initial results ... but then I gained the weight back. Maybe you've had a similar experience with a diet you felt good about.

I tried the low-sugar diet, the one where you consume less than 100 calories worth of sugar per day and make other major changes from the "default" meal plans that most people in our country follow. Same story. The diet worked for a while ... I got some good initial results ... but then I gained the weight back.

I tried Atkins, the low-carb weight-loss plan, and I followed its instructions to the letter. Guess what? It worked for a while ... I got some good results ... but then I gained the weight back.

I tried the Primal diet, which is based on eating foods that so-called "primitive" people would have eaten, thousands of years ago. Leaving aside the premise of the book – I believe human beings are human beings, regardless of what labels people decide to put on them – the result was a familiar one. The diet worked for a while ... I got some good results ... but then I gained the weight back.

I tried the Whole 30 diet, where you build your meal plan around "clean" foods that have no artificial ingredients added. That's actually a very important principle to work toward, one with which I agree whole-heartedly. But as far as the plan itself – the day-by-day instructions I was following so carefully – did it work? No. Whole 30 worked for a while ... I got some good results ... but then I gained the weight back.

I tried a lot of other plans, too, always with the same stressful, morale-shattering result: I gained all the weight back ... sometimes even more weight than I started out with!

Why?

Unable to find the answer to that question, Nadine and I realized that this was the point at which a lot of people simply gave up. But we thought of our family, and we decided I just couldn't do that. So,

> "I gained all the weight back ... sometimes even more weight than I started out with!"

we kept digging. Kept comparing programs. Kept evaluating. Kept comparing and contrasting the plans. Kept asking ourselves – what worked here?

After studying all the major (and minor) diets out there, everything that delivered any kind of positive result, we noticed that they shared some intriguing common ground. Although many of the diets had "secret" reasons why they worked, they had some common ground: certain food choices that were recommended by all of them, the timing of meals and snacks, and an emphasis on exercise.

As we continued our research, we started to find more common ground. We noticed that movement and diet were not the only elements found in all their instructions. There was also an emphasis on proper sleep and hydration.

There was something else, though, which the diets had not picked up on. I knew from my training and experience in soft tissue damage that you need to balance stress on the body and to remove the mental, physical, and structural effects of negative stress. Thanks to prior knowledge and training, I already recognized that diet, exercise, sleep, and hydration were all interconnected. Now I was

THE WAKE-UP CALL

starting to look at how important the whole question of stress was: what it does to the human body, and specifically the effect it has on a weight-loss plan. Stress management, I realized, was something important that I had left out of the equation.

As Nadine and I continued to study diets, exercise, healthy living, and related topics, we came across another important area to consider: We studied the common ground among the oldest living people in the world, their cultural background, and the differences in their life choices. We took all that into account, and a pattern started to form.

The book you are now holding in your hands is the outcome of all our studies, the common ground we identified that connects people who are able to lose weight, live fit, enjoy life, and most important, *stay the course*.

After years of studying different plans, lifestyles, and exercise theories, Nadine and I decided to take on a national program and become certified as nutrition and health coaches. Our training confirmed and reinforced what we had discovered in our initial studies, that in order to lose weight, live fit, and enjoy life, you can't just change what you eat and how you exercise. To lose weight and keep it off, you need to have a comprehensive weight-loss program that encompasses *five* separate elements of your lifestyle ... and changes them all for the better!

Here's what I figured out in my own life: Yes, I needed to lose weight. But I had another problem, an even bigger one, which I had overlooked. My life was out of balance! The fundamental problem I had wasn't the "diets" in and of themselves – the list of foods I was supposed to eat or not eat. The problem was my definition of the word "diet." It didn't go far enough.

REDEFINING THE WORD "DIET"

The moral of this story is: *If you want to diet in a way that keeps the weight off, you can't just look at what you put in your mouth. That's only one-fifth of what dieting really involves.*

By redefining what I meant by the word "diet," I set new priorities and reached my optimal weight of 180 pounds. I tell you that not to impress you, but to inspire you to do what I did: *take action to make sure the weight loss is permanent. The benefits far outweigh the effort.*

The way to make a diet stick is to redefine the definition of diet. It means so much more than just restricting the food we eat, or counting calories, or eating only certain foods. Diet needs to focus on and change five parts of your life, not just one. Maybe that sounds difficult. So did driving a car when you first started doing that! Changing your lifestyle takes practice, yes, but it's doable, and it eventually becomes second nature, just like driving a car. And guess what? It's the *only* approach that works. This is what allowed me to make my 180-degree turn ... and keep the weight off.

Thank God, I was able to turn my car around ... and I was able to keep it heading in the right direction, away from that cliff. During this time, Nadine and I came to appreciate three fundamental truths:

- **We all have a right to good health.** The kind of health disaster I experienced was totally preventable. Not only should it not have happened to me, it shouldn't happen to anyone.

- **This is a mission.** Returning to peak condition and staying in peak condition wasn't just about me. My recovery had to mean something. It had to be part of a larger effort to keep other people from having to go through the hell I had gone through. Now, I am all about making that effort.

- **Balance matters.** To lose weight and keep it off, I had to restore some *balance* to my life. You need to do this too. The human body doesn't operate on one level only; if you want to improve your quality of life in a meaningful, sustainable way – and remember, I had no choice but to do that if I wanted to get off the Wall of Shame – you have to do what I did: take a balanced, holistic approach to the task of living a healthier, happier, and more youthful life in *five different areas*. Specifically, you have to create your own ideal lifestyle in each of those areas ... and then you have to LIVE IT!

If you're wondering what those five different lifestyle areas are ... good. I need you to want to know the answer. And you're almost ready to find out.

There are five things that need to happen consistently if you want to turn your body vehicle around and keep it moving smoothly in the right direction. The five habits you need to build your life around are:

 RECHARGE
Plug in your body's battery and get back to 100% (by getting enough sleep).

 FUEL
Fill your body up with quality food (by eating right).

 DRIVE
Move your body regularly (by actively using it).

 CONNECT
Set your personal destination (by building a sense of purpose and social interaction into your daily life).

 REPAIR
Remove the adverse effects of life on your body (by managing stress effectively).

Skipping one or more of these steps in your daily life leads to big trouble. Your body's vehicle will break down and become diseased or, worse, deceased!

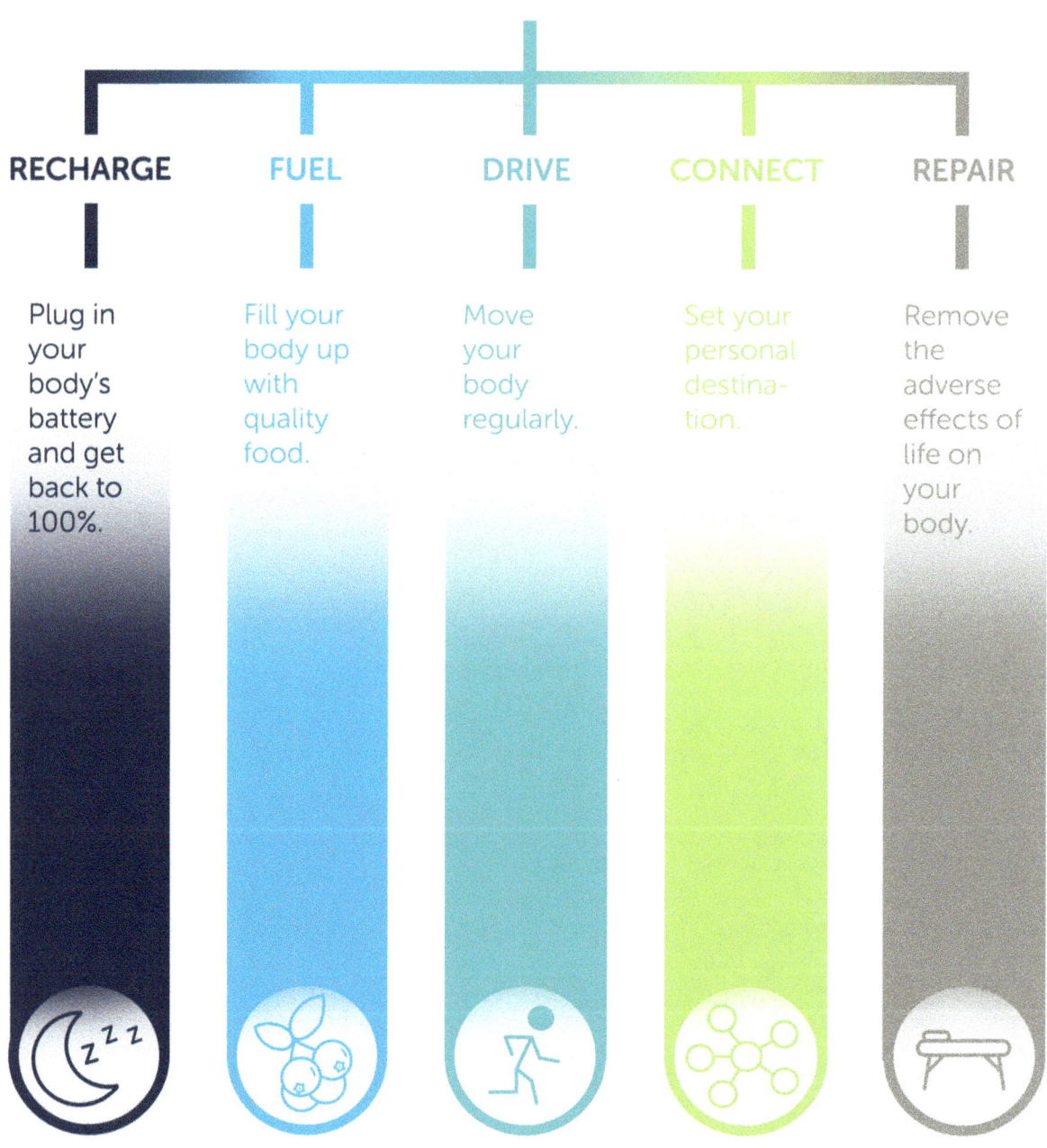

Notice that simply improving the quality and quantity of the food you eat is *not enough*.

I must emphasize this point. This is the reason all those so-called "diet plans" so often fail to deliver sustainable results – people focus only on the stuff they eat, leaving just about everything else out of the equation. It's true, I was eating a lot of crap, in very large portions, for well over a decade ... but I was also neglecting my sleep, my exercise, my social life, and my stress management, in a self-perpetuating downward spiral that darn near killed me. The cumulative impact of all those problems, the lifestyle I had embraced, was what put me at risk. To recover, I needed to address all those areas and choose a different way of living ... not just change my "diet."

A side note: Who really wants to go on a "diet?" Even the word, for most of us, conjures up feelings of being restricted, of being kept from doing what we want to do. Let's face it, dieting doesn't sound fun. In fact, it sounds way too much like dying!

Therefore, don't just diet ... find a plan that changes your life for the good, find a lifestyle that supports you ... a *lifestyle* that's in alignment with the way the human body was designed ... and then LIVE IT!

In the next chapter, I'll share some of the most important takeaways that Nadine and I built into the only diet that actually works ... the diet that's meant to keep you from heading over the same cliff I was racing toward. The only diet that will charge your lifestyle!

LIVE-IT! 180° INSIGHT

I call the system I am sharing with you here **LIVE-IT! 180°**. That's because it's a "live-it," a plan for living, the exact opposite of the type of "diet and exercise plan" that people burn out on after a few weeks. LIVE-IT! 180° is designed to be liberating rather than constricting. If you do it right, which I'm committed to helping you do, it will stick with you over time, so that you too can "do a 180," lose the weight, and keep it off.

Before you read any of that, though, I need you to read this.

THE OTHER AMBULANCE TRIP

One of the things that made that 2012 trip to the emergency room so harrowing for me was the reality that I used to be a paramedic volunteer who supported ambulance teams. I could remember the day that I showed up at a car accident caused by a drunk driver. Everyone on the scene – the police, the other members of the ambulance team

– went out of their way to praise the driver who'd caused the crash. Why? Because he had chosen to swerve his vehicle in such a way that he saved two kids who were strapped into the back of the car he had run into, and because, after the collision, he stumbled out of his own car and extracted the children from the wreckage, saving their lives. However, the crash had killed their mother, who was driving the other vehicle.

Here's my point. The drunk driver's choice to save the kids didn't make him a hero. A real hero would not have got drunk and sat behind the wheel in the first place. I'm willing to bet there was a moment when he heard a voice that said, *Hey, you're making a big mistake.*

The driver ignored that voice – and that choice had consequences. Now he has to live with that mistake for the rest of his life. What would he give to have that moment back?

So, here's the thing. This book is all about choices. I believe that each of us, deep down, knows when we're making a bad choice. It's just a question of whether we're willing to listen to the little voice inside that tells us, quietly but firmly, that we're making a big mistake.

Please bear in mind: The choices we make today are what determine our future.

Everything that follows in this book is here to help you make choices that support you ... as opposed to choices that are likely to send you hurtling into a future you really, really don't want (the emergency room, for instance). I can't make any of those choices for you. But if you let me, I can guide and support you as you make them, because I've been down this road before. I can help you learn to listen to that little voice, the one I ignored for over a decade. And I can tell you where the nastiest twists and turns are on the road, so you can make the best decisions – the decisions that keep you moving forward safely. I can help you to get where you need to go, where you were meant to go.

Shall we make that journey together?

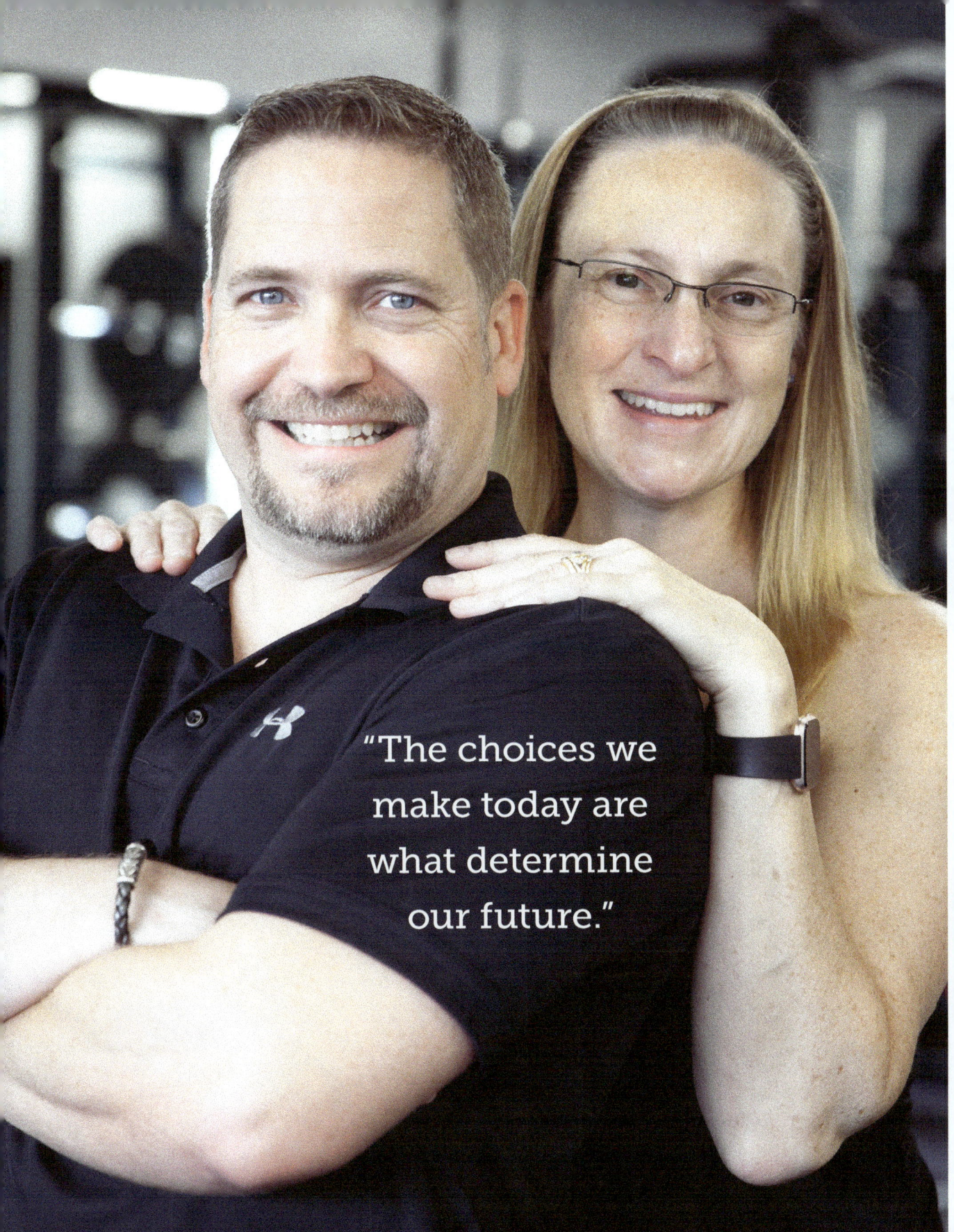

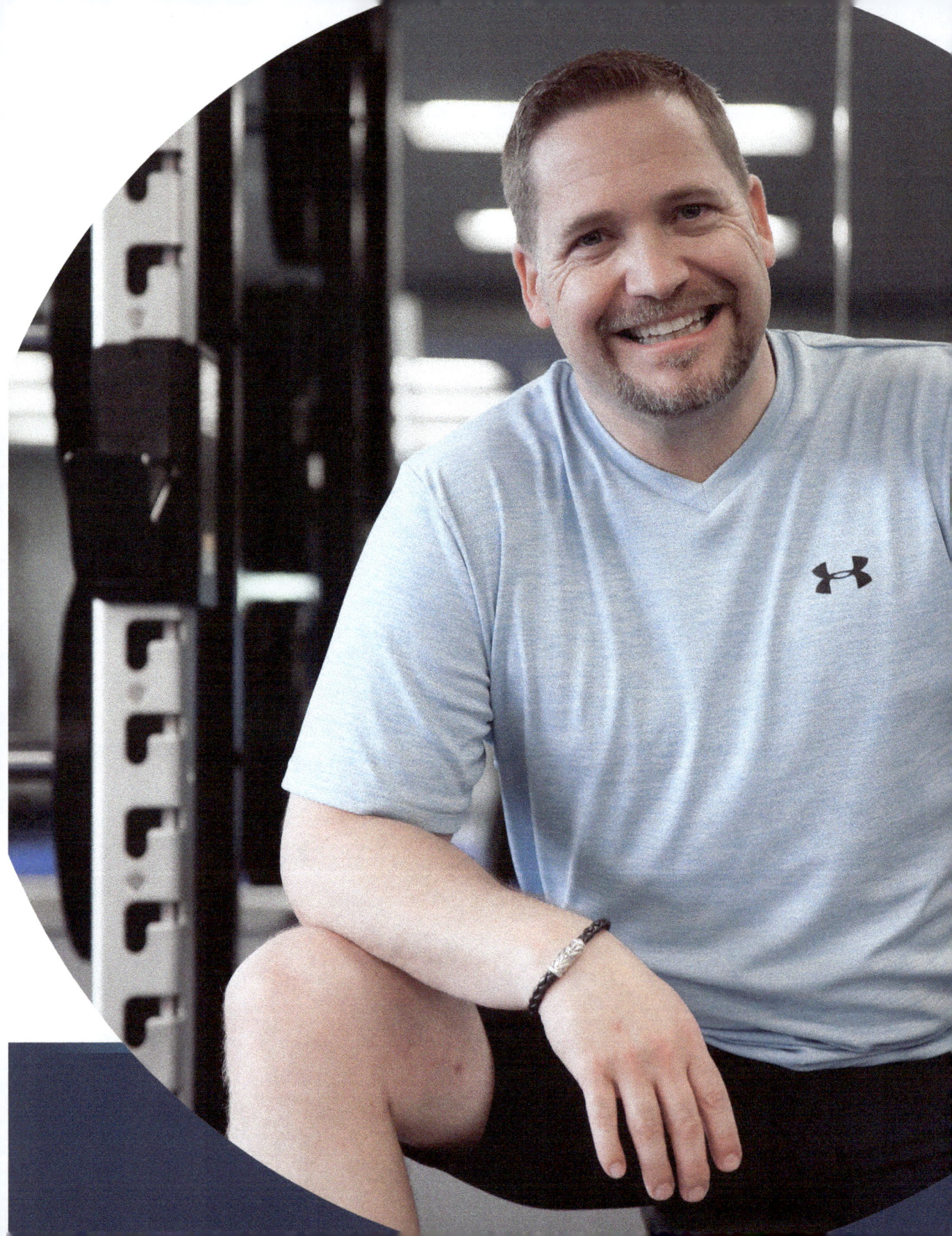

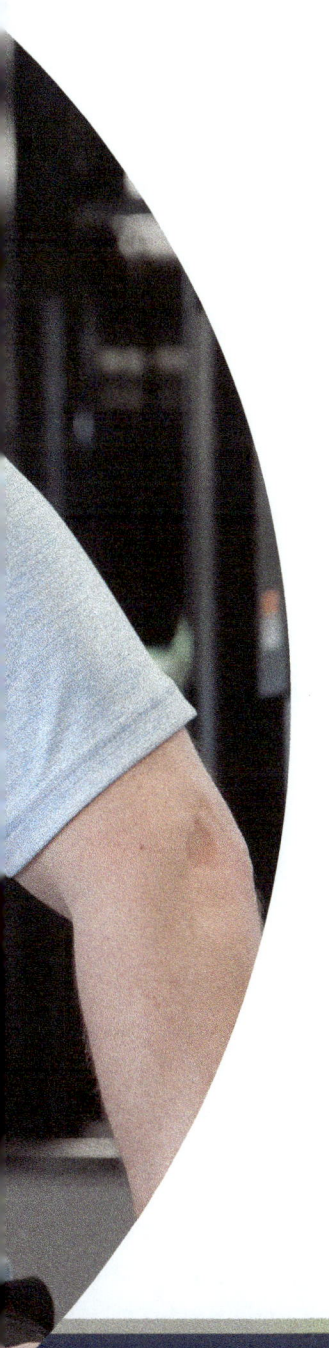

MY REQUEST TO YOU

After my doctor showed me the Wall of Shame, I knew I had to turn my life around. To use the term he used, I knew it was time for me to do a 180. Maybe it's time for you to do one, too.

As you now know, I tried all kinds of different "diets" as I figured out how to make my turnaround ... and I compared what I learned about them to what I already knew about the many different "fitness plans" that are out there. Here's what I noticed: Some of these plans work – for a while, depending on the level of support and coaching you chose to build into your routine – and some of them don't.

Among the ones that definitely *don't* work are the plans that suggest you can create and sustain rapid weight loss in just a few weeks ... by making a few radical, short-term changes in menu and exercise.

Some of these plans, for instance, urge you to cut your calorie intake way, way down for a brief period – seven days, fourteen days, twenty-one days – to almost dangerous levels. The problem with this kind of crash-and-burn approach is that the weight you lose will always come back with a vengeance when you start eating "normally" again ... which, of course, you will.

This brings us to my first piece of advice for you: **Please don't follow those "diets."** They will only waste your precious time, and they may actually hurt you.

THREE BIG LIFE LESSONS

One big thing Nadine and I learned from my 180° journey is that **none of us need a "diet plan" like that.** What we really need is support from a coach and/or accountability partner as we develop good habits that we live out every day – naturally – in harmony with our body's own Intelligent Design. You and I will be talking a lot more about this term, Intelligent Design, in the pages the follow. For now, just understand that, once we bring our habits into line with our body's natural design, once we reinforce those habits over time, they can become our way of life. They can become the *new* habits we live by, as opposed to the old habits that point our car toward the cliff edge.

But ... new habits always need a reason. Which brings me to the second big thing I learned during this journey: **When you have the education and the motivation, your habits will change for the better ... and positive results will come!** In other words: The more I learned about what actually worked, the more motivated I was to implement it in my own life. So, this book, and the **LIVE-IT! 180°** system it outlines, is meant to give you all the education you need to get motivated to take action that will help you lose weight and keep it off.

The third big thing I learned from my journey back from the abyss is that **what I accomplished in my own life was meaningless if I didn't share it with other people.** I realized that my mission was to help other people create the same kind of turnaround. We all need a life coach or accountability partner to keep us on track. I want this book to begin the process of building that kind of accountability into your world, so you can lose the weight and keep it off ... and then maybe help someone else to do the same.

To begin with, I will be your coach – right here on the page, which is the perfect place to start. In the next chapter, I'll give you more background on your own astonishing Intelligent Design. In chapters Four through Eight, I'll be sharing, not a single set of rules for you to follow, but multiple options – Good, Better, and Best – in each of the five critical areas of life that we'll be looking at: **RECHARGE, FUEL, DRIVE, CONNECT,** and **REPAIR.**

That's the eight-week system I'll be sharing with you, as your new lifestyle coach. That's the **LIVE-IT! 180°** system in a nutshell. It's all about keeping your body and your life in alignment with your own Intelligent Design ... by making good, conscious choices.

It's going to be up to you which of those options you pick, how you customize them to your world, and how you put them into practice. As your coach, I'm going to help you get crystal-clear on the kinds of choices that will help you to turn your life around–and do a 180.

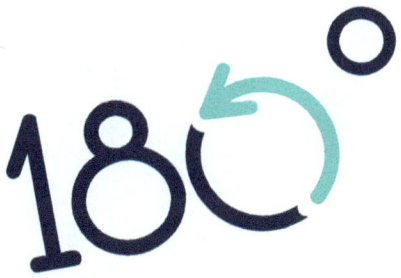

By the way, that number 180 is important for another reason: it breaks down my promise to you:

Adopt just ONE simple, easy-to-implement set of habits per week ...

... for EIGHT straight weeks ...

... and you will be able to lose weight (and keep it off), live fit, and enjoy life, with ZERO regrets.

A REQUEST

This book is built on the following very simple principle: Every choice we make determines our future. The corollary of that principle is equally simple: We all need to make the right choices, the choices that will give us a 180° lifestyle shift when we're headed in the wrong direction. With this book, I am here to support you, coach you, and provide you with both the accountability and the education you need to get motivated to make better lifestyle choices. Guidance and support can also be found at our web site, Liveit180.com.

So, here's my request: Will you let me be your coach?

If your answer is yes ... if you're ready to make **LIVE-IT! 180°** a reality ... if you're ready to plan and live your life in a way that allows you to lose weight and stay healthy, it's time for us to move on to the next chapter.

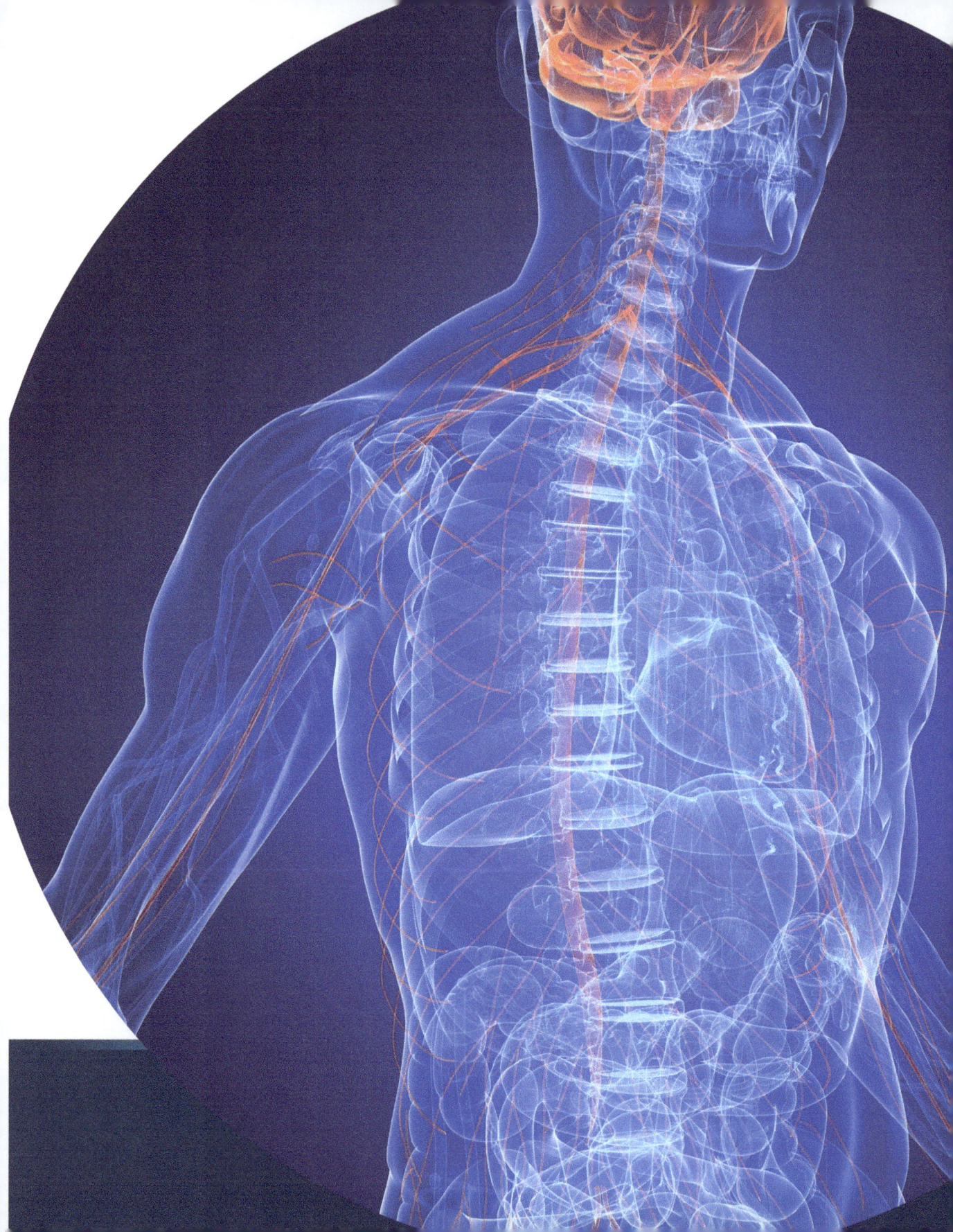

INTELLIGENT DESIGN

3

The book you're holding in your hands is the fulfilment of my life's passion, conviction, and belief, which can be summarized as follows:

- The human body presents clear evidence of Intelligent Design.

- This Design didn't happen by chance or because of a Big Bang, millions of years ago.

- We will all live happier, healthier, and more youthful lives, at our optimum weight, if we maintain our bodies in accordance with the manufacturer's (simple) guidelines.

Personally, I'm content to call this higher power God, though I know some will contest the existence of God or call what I'm talking about by many other names. They may be convinced (because of a man-made science, which has its limits) that we came by this body as a result of millions of years of evolution, by chance. Call God by any name you want, or use any theory you desire, but for the purpose of this book, I am going to refer to Him as the Designer. What matters to me most is not what you *call* this power, or what you believe, but that you recognize your body is unique in creation, that it has an Intelligent Design that is begging you, warning you, pleading with you, to learn how to *respond* to it.

What you'll find in this book is a series of ideas for tapping into, and acting on, the Intelligent Design of the remarkable machine we've all been given for the time we're here on earth – our own body. This machine is, quite literally, a miracle: a self-repairing, self-correcting entity that will operate at peak performance levels for each of us for many decades ... if only we learn to recognize its "warning lights" and avoid the mistake of failing to respond to them.

Fortunately, the Designer has made recognizing the warnings easy. All we need to do is learn to *listen* to what the miraculous machine is trying to tell us. Take a cellular call from your body!

Just think. If your car's dashboard started flashing a whole bunch warning lights, wouldn't you stop and get whatever it was warning you to fix taken care of? Of course you would. Why? Because if you didn't, the car could stop working.

LIVE-IT! 180° INSIGHT

The human body is a miraculous, self-correcting, self-repairing entity that will operate at peak performance levels for each of us for many decades ... if only we learn to recognize and respond to its "warning lights."

In this chapter, I'll share two core concepts that will help you in later chapters as you move into the habit of recognizing, understanding, and heeding those "warning lights" incorporated into the design of your miraculous body. Before I share these concepts, let me invite you to consider the following fact. To paraphrase Thomas Jefferson, it's a truth I hold to be self-evident.

YOU ARE NOT AN ACCIDENT

The universe is not an accident. The Earth is not an accident. And neither are you.

I believe all of us are here on purpose, by Design. I believe none of us is here because of random chance. We are here for a reason. We are part of a system that, on both the small and large scales, is too perfect to have come about as the result of "coincidence."

The rate at which the universe expands, must be (and is) delicately balanced to incredible precision in order for it to exist. If the universe expanded more quickly than this delicate balance dictates, matter would expand too quickly for the formation of stars, planets, and galaxies. If it expanded more slowly, the universe would collapse before stars could form. The Designer has established the perfect speed for the universe.

Similarly, the Designer has expertly encoded literally billions of chunks of information within the structure of our DNA molecules. We take this encoding for granted or, perhaps, don't even

> *"The universe is not an accident. The Earth is not an accident. And neither are you."*

realize it exists at such a microscopic level. When coding of that complexity takes place within a software program, none of us has any doubt that the coding the computer runs for us is the result of conscious, manmade intent. Nobody would argue that such software could materialize on its own or by chance. So why do we ignore the even more complex design within the molecules of our own bodies? It's a far more intricate design then any software program, so why do we think it could have "just happened" by chance or accident?

What about the reality that the earth's very design parallels our own – that approximately 70% of the earth's surface is covered with water and approximately 70% of a healthy human adult's body is composed of water? Isn't such a parallel something more than coincidence? Isn't it possible that this parallel is evidence of some close, *intentional* connection between our own Design and that of the planet we live on?

If you're willing to at least consider accepting this Intelligent Design concept ... then you and I are ready to explore two of the most important Design features within the miraculous machine that is your body. I'll share them with you by means of two metaphors: **The Vehicle** and **The Orchestra**.

Put these two metaphors together, and they'll help you to learn to recognize the "alarms and warning lights" that the Designer has built into your extraordinary machine, act appropriately, and support your body as it restores its own natural balance.

The Vehicle

Intelligent Design has given you a miraculous state-of-the art, high-performance vehicle; one that not only flashes warning signals when something is about to go wrong, but also *self-repairs* as you drive it – if you do what the warning lights tell you to do. Pretty remarkable, right? But there's a catch.

If you consistently *don't* pay attention to the warning lights ... if you make a habit of *not* doing what the manufacturer recommends ... if you do the *opposite* of what the warning lights are telling you to do and you keep that up for long enough ... the car will break down and may even stop working altogether. It's the only vehicle you're ever going to have ... and you just destroyed your ride!

You have been given only one Intelligently Designed body. Take care of it.

The moral: What we put into our Vehicle matters, how we drive our Vehicle matters, and the warning signals our Vehicle flashes matter too. If a car you can buy has such a deep level of complexity and it's man-made, how much more complex is your Intelligently Designed human body?

How important is that cellular call coming in as you drive, warning you that you're approaching a danger point? How important is that warning sign you see flashing on the dashboard? Very important. Take the call! Heed the warnings! Or you'll suffer dire consequences ... not the least of which is extra weight you're not designed to carry around.

Actually, our body is even more complex than a vehicle. In fact, it's so Intelligently Designed that no single piece of equipment can compare to it. Which brings me to my second metaphor.

> "You have been given only one Intelligently Designed body. Take care of it."

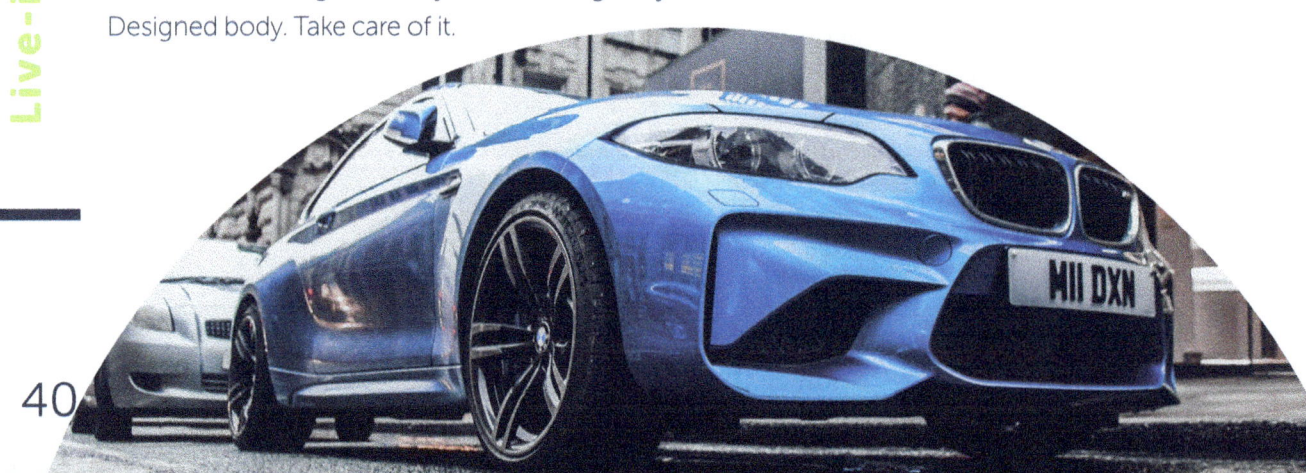

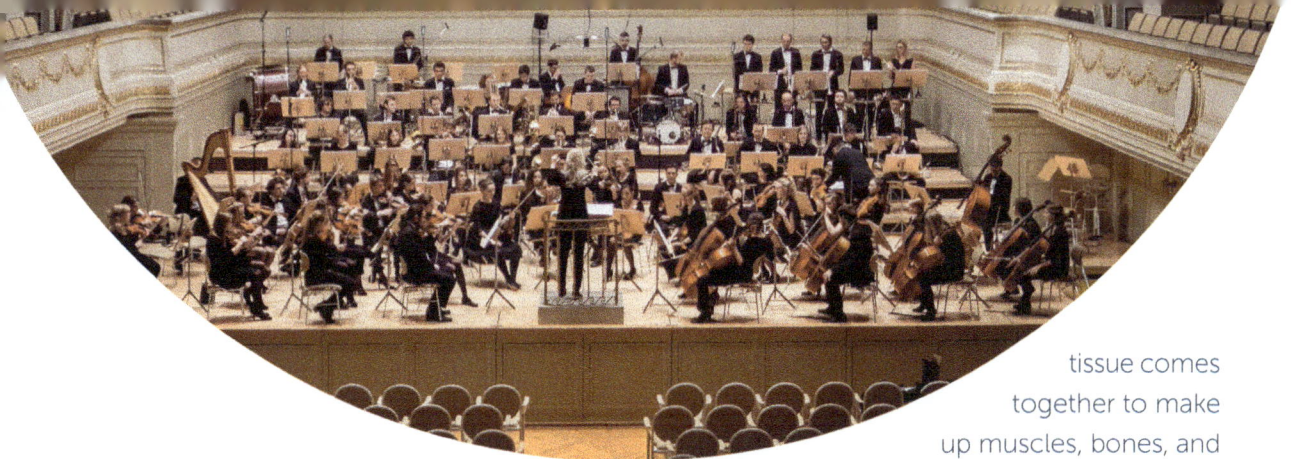

The Orchestra

To help you understand how your body resembles a symphony orchestra, I need to give you an idea of just how many different levels you operate on. Most of us don't realize how intricate and precise and complex our own bodies really are!

The Designer used over seven billion billion billion atoms – that's a seven followed by 27 zeros – to create you. The Designer combined those atoms to form roughly 20,000,000,000,000,000,000,000,000 (twenty septillion) molecules.

Among those molecules is the DNA molecule, the masterpiece of Intelligent Design. Each DNA molecule is structured in such a way as to contain the entire genetic code necessary to generate and/or regenerate every single one of the 37.2 trillion cells in our body.

Now, these cells are highly specialized, and they show up in lots of different forms, from blood to soft tissue to fingernails to brain matter to bones to hair.

All of that is a result of DNA telling your cells – the building blocks of your body – what to do! Your cells come together to make up tissue and your tissue comes together to make up muscles, bones, and organs. All your muscles and bones make up your skeletal and movement system. Your organs work together to make up your breathing or respiratory system, cardiovascular system, endocrine system, digestion, elimination, and central nervous system, etc. Please remember that no matter how the building blocks are formed, *You are, at your foundation, a cellular being.* Every single physical part of you, without exception, is made of cells. And the health of your cells determines the quality of your life.

By Intelligent Design, your body used your trillions of cells to create this amazing interplay of organs or, as we call it here, instruments. The instruments each have a part to play, just like the instruments in a symphony orchestra. And their performance is *you*.

Maybe you're wondering – what's holding it all together? What acts as the Conductor in this amazing symphony orchestra?

That's an important question. Before I answer it, though, let me go back to the cellular level and share one more vitally important insight with you about the cells that are the building blocks of your body:

LIVE-IT! 180° INSIGHT

When it comes to your body, the micro affects the macro. It's all connected.

Your body operates at a cellular level. This means that your cellular health determines the health of your tissues, your organs, your various life-support systems, and your body as a whole. **It all comes down to how well you take care of your cells.**

The health of your cells, in turn, is determined by:

- How well you sleep

- What you eat

- What kind of physical movement you do

- The quality of your relationships with others

- The way you handle stress

Your daily decisions in each of these five areas – the five areas of life that make up the **LIVE-IT! 180° System** – affect you on a fundamental, *cellular* level ... which affects your tissues ... which affects your organs ... which affects your systems ... which affects the quality of the "orchestra performance" that is your life.

Problems like cancer and diabetes and high cholesterol don't just happen. They are the result of the *decisions* we make in each of the five areas of **LIVE-IT! 180°**.

Everything you do to your body's cells affects the quality of the orchestra's performance.

THE CONDUCTOR

Believe it or not, the various systems in your body constantly communicate with each other. They coordinate their work seamlessly, making sure that your organs don't overwork or underwork, guaranteeing that every organ in your body supports the work of every other organ. The systems operate on their own and at the same time are entirely dependent on each other. It's a truly amazing performance. Who's in charge of holding it all together? Who makes sure all that harmonious communication happens? The Conductor, of course.

On a technical level, scientists will tell you that the process by which all the body's systems are kept in harmony is something called homeostasis, which is a function of the autonomic nervous system. That's the "autopilot" part of your brain that controls body systems like blood pressure, heart rate, respiration, water balance, and body temperature without your conscious thought. While all of that is true, I believe this technical answer doesn't go far enough.

I believe the Conductor of your body's great symphony is your very essence, spirit, or soul, controlling your *Intelligent Design in its active mode*.

Your Intelligent Design has two aspects to it that are important to understand. It has an active mode, when you are in control of the symphony, and an autopilot mode, when your assistant conductor by Design takes over. This interchanging active to autopilot mode in action is the essence of who you are. Some people call this essence the soul; others call it the life force. Whatever you call it, it's what is keeping everything working in harmony even as you read these words.

Right now, as you read this, your heart is pumping, and your lungs are breathing, and your visual cortex is processing tens of thousands of signals. All these things are happening independently, but at the same time, they are part of a powerful, coordinated symphony of instruments playing in perfect harmony.

Each individual cell of your body has its own unique piece of the symphony to play in this performance. Through active and autopilot mode, you use the Intelligent Design body to match all the pieces together and lead the orchestra in a way

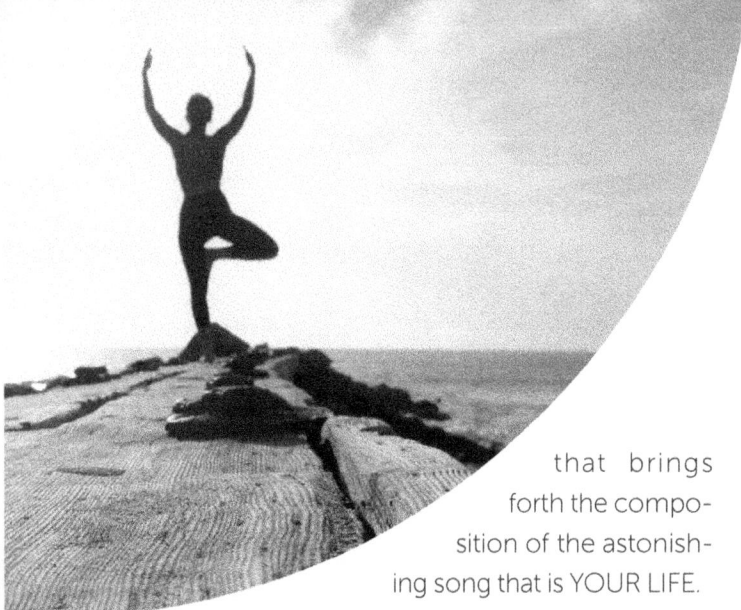

...that brings forth the composition of the astonishing song that is YOUR LIFE.

I believe our job as human beings is pretty simple: **Be the active Conductor of your life and respond to the autopilot's warning lights.** I wrote this book to help you learn how to pick up the Conductor's stick and let the Intelligent Design direct the body's miraculous ability to work in harmony ... and remain in harmony.

Unfortunately, it's easier than you might think to get out of harmony and lose rhythm as the conductor. Let me give you a personal example that will illustrate exactly what I mean.

ARE YOU SABOTAGING THE INTELLIGENTLY DESIGNED AUTOPILOT CONDUCTOR?

Earlier on in this book, I mentioned that I had a major health crisis, culminating in an agonizing case of kidney stones. Now, traditional Western medicine would be likely to tell someone in my situation that the problem was my kidney stones. In fact, the problem was me not listening to the warning signs produced by Intelligent Design. I was sabotaging the Intelligently Designed autopilot Conductor.

LIVE-IT! 180° gives you five ways you can make it easier for the active and autopilot Conductors to guide the interdependent, codependent systems that make up your Intelligently Designed human body – your orchestra. In the months before I knew I *had* a "kidney stone problem," I had been in "sabotage the autopilot Conductor" mode in four of those five areas.

I was not sleeping well. I was eating junk food that wasn't what my body needed (and not drinking enough water). I was getting virtually no exercise. I was under constant stress, and I wasn't dealing with it well. The only thing I had going for me, if you're keeping score at home, is that my social life and family life were strong. But I was criminally neglecting those other four areas ... and as a result, the orchestra was playing further and further out of tune, despite the autopilot Conductor's best efforts to bring me back into balance.

I could have noticed what was happening, but I didn't. I ignored the increasingly off-key notes – like pain in my side and back and below my ribs; pain that came in waves and fluctuated in intensity; pain when I urinated; nausea and vomiting. That was the sound of my body – my orchestra – trying to tell me something. But I didn't listen. I waited for it to get better.

Do you know what was happening inside me while I was ignoring the increasing tunelessness of my orchestra? My autopilot Conductor was trying to fix the damage I'd done to my body.

Because of my neglect, my body had become dangerously acidic. Intelligent Design – the Conductor – was in crisis management mode. The autopilot Conductor tried to restore my low calcium levels by robbing calcium from my bones. It was trying to bring it back from that acidic state to a safe, neutral level. One byproduct of that effort was that little calcium balls built up over time in my kidneys – and the only way to get rid of them was to pee them out, an excruciating experience I wouldn't wish on anyone. This was all because I kept sabotaging my own Conductor and was too oblivious to notice. In the chapters that follow, I'll share the **LIVE-IT! 180°** system I used to bring myself back into balance.

REDUCTIONISM: What does that mean?

Western medicine will tell you I had a kidney stone problem. That's because Western medicine does not take a holistic approach. It looks at the human body through a lens called *reductionism.*

Basically, reductionism means doctors try to reduce whatever health question you've got down to the most basic part and to fix that component, rather than looking at the body as a whole. The problem with this approach is that it attacks the symptoms, rather than addressing the cause. I didn't have a kidney stone problem. I had an imminent-orchestral-failure problem, because I had been ignoring the out-of-tune notes and the warning lights for months.

This book hopes to make it easier for you to address the *causes* behind the most common health problems. It's here to help you get your body back into the self-monitoring, self-healing phase where all the autopilot conductor has to do is point the baton and bring everything back into sync. All the systems in your body are interconnected at a cellular level. They operate both independently and codependently, seamlessly connecting with each other, by Intelligent Design. If you disrupt the balance, ignore the off-key notes, and damage the cells, guess what? You're sabotaging yourself – and the entire orchestra!

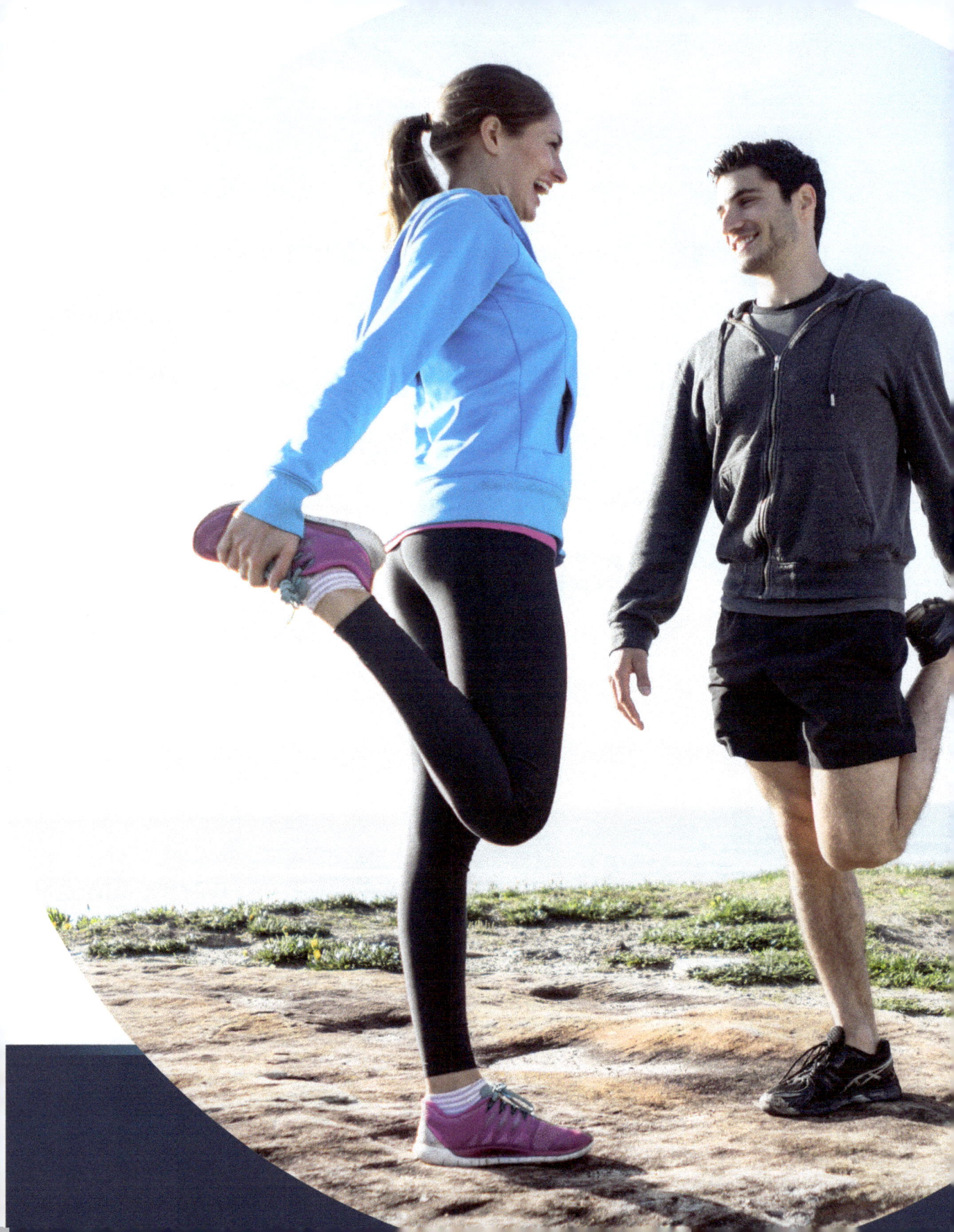

A BRIEF OVERVIEW OF LIVE-IT! 180°

4

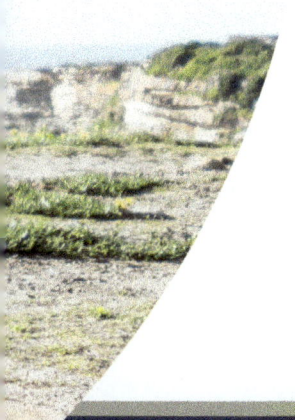

If, God forbid, you were diagnosed with cancer tomorrow morning, the American Cancer Society would have all kinds of great advice for you and suggest that you make numerous lifestyle changes. They would tell you that by following that advice, you would substantially increase your chances of living a longer, happier life. And you know what? Most of that advice would also be extremely beneficial for people who *don't* have cancer!

Which brings up an interesting question: **Why should you have to wait until you're dying to start to live?**

Maybe you're wondering, If I don't have cancer, or some other serious disease, why should I consider *any* kind of lifestyle change? Why not keep doing what I'm already doing? Why not stay inside my comfort zone?

Because, if you're like most of the people reading this book, you're probably in the same situation I was in when I was ramping my way up to a major kidney-stone emergency. Alarms are going off. Lights on the dashboard are flashing. Bells are ringing. Each and every one of us who notices these warnings has to decide: Am I going to respond or am I going to ignore this?

The correct answer to that question, by the way, is RESPOND. If the emergency light on the dashboard flashes, you pull over (if you're smart). If the fire alarm is going off, you get out of the building. And if your body is telling you there's a problem, you listen and take action! If your orchestra is out of tune or out of sync, you need to address it or the song of your life will have no harmony.

When you're overweight, when you don't have the energy you should have, when you're having trouble making it up a flight of stairs, when your body aches or has unexplained pains, *that's an alarm going off.* And right now, your body is telling you exactly what it needs you to do to deal with those alarms. The problem is, most of us don't listen very well. We ignore the alarms, imagining that they'll go away.

That's a mistake. If you choose to ignore the extra weight, the sluggishness, the reduced mobility, or any of the other flashing red lights on your dashboard, *you will compromise your body's entire, interconnected system.* You will find yourself on a spiraling downward path.

> "If you choose to ignore the extra weight, the sluggishness, the reduced mobility, or any of the other flashing red lights on your dashboard, you will find yourself on a spiraling downward path."

LIVE-IT! 180° INSIGHT

LIVE-IT! 180° makes it easier for you to notice, listen to, and respond to the alarms your body sets off when it's out of balance. LIVE-IT! 180° honors your body's own Intelligent Design for losing weight, living fit, enjoying life, respecting the holistic nature of your body, and sharing simple best practices that support you in five equally critical, interrelated areas of your daily life. It provides you with Good, Better, and Best tactics for optimizing the way you:

 RECHARGE your body's battery (by getting enough sleep).

 FUEL your body (by eating right).

 DRIVE your body regularly (by actively moving and exercising).

 CONNECT your body to a destination (by building a sense of purpose and social interaction into your daily life).

 REPAIR your body from life's effects (by managing stress effectively).

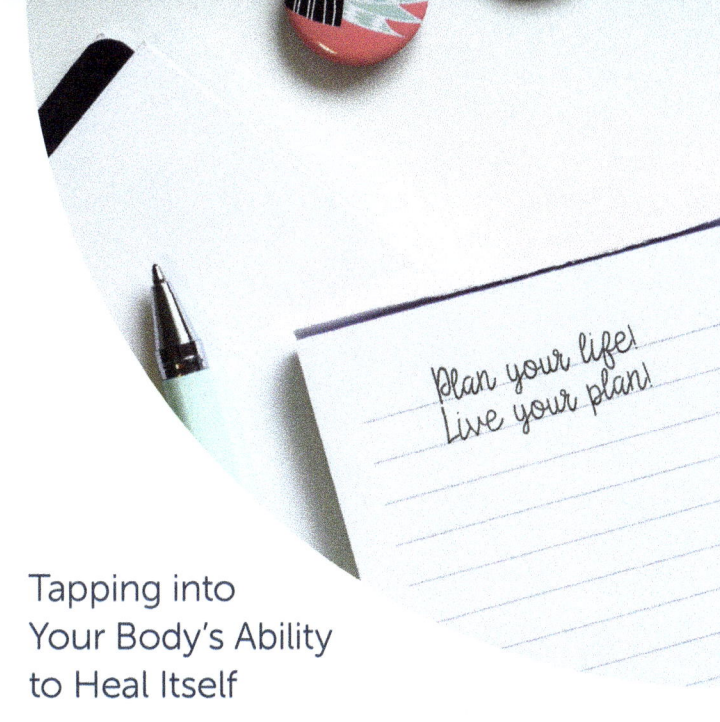

Tapping into Your Body's Ability to Heal Itself

In order to make choices that are life-changing and have lasting positive results, you need to develop lifestyle habits that tap into the genius of your body's Intelligent Design. **LIVE-IT! 180°** provides the *education* and *motivation* that enable you to develop these habits, leveraging the astonishing self-healing capacity of the miracle that is your human body.

You can achieve so much if you leverage this: your ideal weight, ideal stamina, ideal hormone balance, reduced inflammation, an optimal functioning of your immune system, and a profound enhancement of your personal well-being. In short, you can become the "you" you were designed to be. If losing weight, living fit, and enjoying life is your goal, **LIVE-IT! 180°** is perfect for you.

LIVE-IT! 180° is not about following the latest food fad. It's not about killing yourself in the gym. It's not something you should only do if your health

A BRIEF OVERVIEW OF LIVE-IT! 180°

49

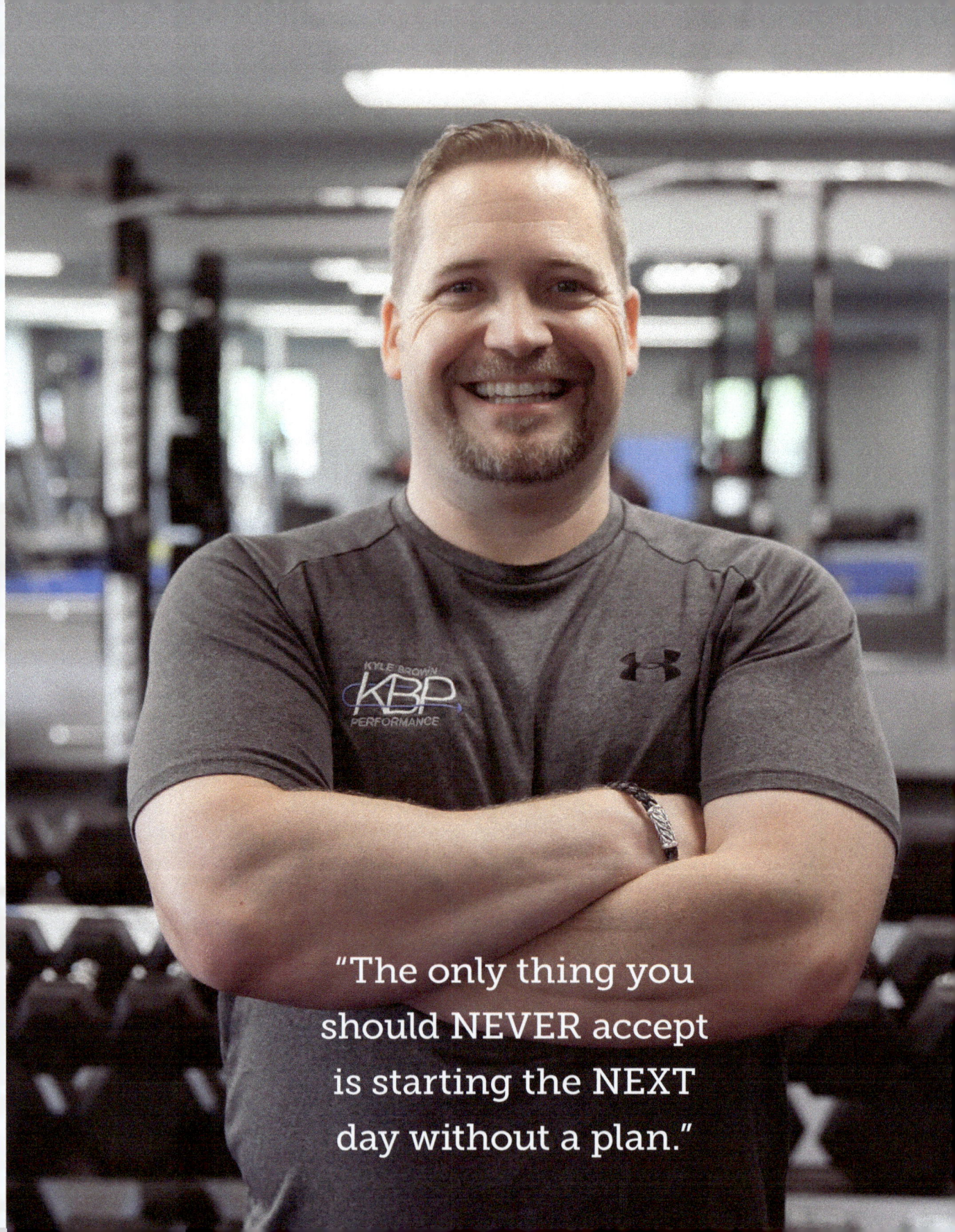

deteriorates and triggers your body's alarm system. It's not about waiting until you're sick to start living healthier. It's about acting on the reality that your body already knows how to take care of itself.

Take a Cellular Call from Your Body ... Before It's Too Late!

Listening to our Intelligently Designed bodies means overcoming some existing patterns of behavior, some of them deeply ingrained. Why? Because over the years, we've been trained to *not* listen to our bodies. It's taken a lifetime to get where you are today. Change can happen, but not overnight. When you develop new habits, which align with your Intelligent Design, great things can happen.

LIVE-IT! 180° is a simple, accessible system that teaches us what our bodies are saying and shows us how to develop life-changing habits that enable us to restore our perfect weight, live fit, and enjoy our life. LIVE-IT! 180° attunes you to the reality that this can be achieved through a series of planned, daily choices. It's an opportunity to plan your life and live your plan.

Don't put this off. Don't assume the alarms you are hearing will take care of themselves. *Take action ... starting right now. The four most deadly words are: "It will go away."* I speak from personal experience on this point.

"The four most deadly words are: 'It will go away'."

The Five Critical Habits (5 Pillars of Health)

There are five critical habits your body needs to develop in order to maintain optimum health. Let's look at each of them in a little more depth.

 You have to RECHARGE your body's battery and get back to 100% (by getting enough sleep)

Getting enough of the right kind of sleep is fundamental to achieving health, happiness, youthfulness, and energy.

 You have to FUEL your body up with quality food (by eating right)

Giving the body the right fuel, in the right quantities, is essential to balancing our hormones, eliminating inflammation, attaining our perfect weight, settling our immune system, and feeling good.

 You have to DRIVE your body regularly (by moving and exercising)

Moving strengthens our muscle tissue and builds stamina. It provides flexibility, aids in the elimination of toxins, helps us to assimilate nutrients, and makes us happier.

You have to CONNECT your body to a destination you want to reach (by building a sense of purpose and social interaction into your daily life)

Connecting with others in person gives purpose and meaning to our lives. It gives us a reason to live and stimulates our brains as well as enhancing our mood.

 And you have to REPAIR your body from the effects of life (by managing stress effectively)

De-stressing from the inevitable challenges of life enables us to live younger and happier. Removing the plaque of stress from our bodies is crucial to living lives that are healthier, happier, and more youthful.

Again: LIVE-IT! 180° is not just a "diet." It's a weight loss system that will change your lifestyle, a habit-driven way of living that educates and motivates. It provides a series of simple, implementable, escalating action items you can adopt over time to reclaim and address your body's natural priorities according to your Intelligent Design. **LIVE-IT! 180° works as a sustainable weight-loss plan because it gives your Intelligently Designed body exactly what it needs in each of those five areas.**

> "Don't just plan your life. LIVE-IT!"

By creating a new daily routine, you can unlock the self-cleansing, self-regulating, self-repairing genius of the greatest piece of Intelligent Design on planet Earth: the human body. **Don't just plan your life. LIVE-IT!**

Warning:
You Can't Do "Part of This"

A key aspect of LIVE-IT! 180° is its *non-negotiable integrity*. That means all five habits are interconnected and interdependent. Remember the orchestra? It has many components: instruments, musicians, music, conductors, and so on. If you are missing any one piece of it, it wouldn't be complete. It would sound wrong. If you're committed to doing **LIVE-IT! 180°**, you must commit to making daily progress in *all five* areas.

This is an extremely important point. If I'm eating the best stuff in the world, in the optimal quantities, at exactly the right times, but I'm not sleeping well, not moving, not connected with others, and not dealing effectively with the stress in my life, guess what? I'm still going to have huge problems, and I'm not going to lose weight in a sustainable way.

And if I'm getting a great workout every day, but I'm only eating overprocessed "ghost food," not getting a good night's sleep, not maintaining healthy relationships with others, and constantly overstressed, it doesn't matter how good my workout is. I'm living a life that's out of balance.

Most of us are way, way out of balance. Not only that: Most of us are either ignoring the consequences of being out of balance or trying to mask the resulting health issues by taking prescription medicines.

If you just keep masking the issues with medicine, you're never going to cure the problem. You're just going to keep masking them. If you maintain that cycle, it can lead not just to long-term obesity, but to other major problems, including cancer, heart disease, liver shutdown, diabetes, kidney failure, and, you guessed it... death.

So, I am asking you to make a personal commitment, right now, to undertake the *entire* LIVE-IT! 180° System... just as it's laid out in these pages.

"What if I Don't Follow Through?"

Let me promise you something ahead of time: There are going to be times when you fall off the wagon. That's okay. I fall off the wagon all the time. Here's my commitment to you: In the pages that follow, you will get everything you need to create a simple, personalized **LIVE-IT! 180°** routine that you can *enjoy* implementing every single day and revise over time to match your personal living situation. But, *there are going to be times when you don't fulfill the plan*. I accept that up-front, and so should you. The only thing you should *never* accept is starting the *next* day without a plan. If you fall of the wagon, make sure you jump back on the very next day. Make that your commitment to yourself. Sound fair?

One day in which you don't follow a plan can mushroom into a week without following a plan, then a month, and then three months. Pretty soon you're looking at a lifetime without following a plan, which is how most people live. I guarantee that is not where you want to be.

LIVE-IT! 180° INSIGHT

Once you're on the wagon and you're going from point A to point B, it's likely you're going to fall off. Here's the secret to success: You want to hop *right back on the wagon*, just as soon as you notice you slip off. Otherwise, the walk to point B is going to be very long and very hard!

Don't beat yourself up. Don't spend precious time and energy dramatizing whatever it was that went wrong. All that drama does is increase your stress levels, which perpetuates the cycle. Just notice what happened, set up what you want to do the next day, and follow it.

Remember: This is a marathon, not a sprint. Put your practice into place. Live your plan!

So: Is the song of your life in harmony ... right now? Are you happy, healthy, and living younger ... right now? If not, it's time to take action. You are the master conductor of your life. Pick up the conductor's baton and start leading your orchestra – and playing your song. It's time to plan your life and live your plan. It's time to **LIVE-IT!**

Take Action! Here's How to Start LIVE-IT! 180°

Each of the chapters that follow gives you an in-depth breakdown of each core element of **LIVE-IT! 180°**, along with Good, Better, and Best daily practices to help you form your own daily, personalized **LIVE-IT! 180°** routine. As you read each chapter you will begin designing your own **LIVE-IT! 180°** lifestyle by identifying the daily habits that work best for you. Then, in Chapter Ten, I'll coach you through the key choices that will make your first eight **LIVE-IT! 180°** weeks a joyous and vibrantly successful experience – the beginning of a whole new way of life.

"OKAY – BUT WHAT CAN I DO RIGHT NOW?"

Glad you asked. Fortunately, you don't need to wait until you've finished this book to get started. You can jump in right now. You are the master conductor of your **LIVE-IT! 180°** lifestyle ... because you are making the choices.

On the next page are some basic examples of how to get started with **LIVE-IT! 180°**.

These are only basic examples, but they are all good places to start. Remember: With LIVE-IT! 180°, the power lies in your ability to *personalize* your own daily routine!

LIVE-IT! 180° TIP

For in-depth help and guidance on how to customize your **LIVE-IT! 180°** lifestyle, check out Liveit180.com – so we can take our coaching relationship to the next level.

ACCOUNTABILITY

Accountability is a key aspect of **LIVE-IT! 180°**. Making yourself accountable to another person helps to keep you on track and motivated, especially on days you just don't feel like staying the course. An accountability partner will greatly

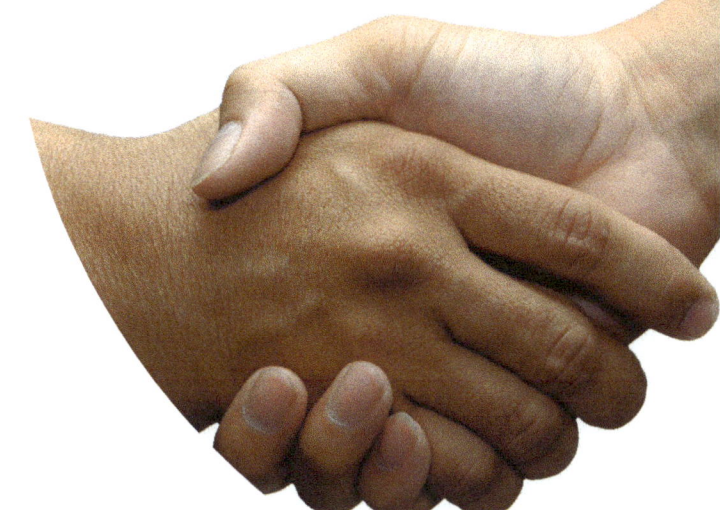

enhance your ability to succeed in all elements of **LIVE-IT! 180°**. Choose wisely, though, as the wrong person can also distract you and keep you from making progress. Remember: Some days may be tougher than others to stick to your **LIVE-IT! 180°** lifestyle. Keeping yourself accountable to a partner who shares your desire to change will help you succeed in creating a happier, healthier, and younger lifestyle!

THE LIVE-IT! 180° HOUSE PLAN

 ### RECHARGE
Get seven and a half hours of uninterrupted sleep every night.

 ### FUEL
Drink half your bodyweight in ounces of water. (For example, a person who weighs 200 pounds should drink 100 ounces of water each day.) At each meal, only eat until you are 80% full. Make sure to include protein, veggies, and a "good" fat, such as avocados, olives, chia seeds, coconut, coconut oil, flaxseeds, or almonds. (We'll get into the more detail about "good" fats a little later in the book.)

 ### DRIVE
Get out and walk for between 15 and 30 minutes each day.

 ### CONNECT
Each day, spend between five and ten minutes connecting with a loved one or friend over the phone or in person.

 ### REPAIR
Each day, take a five-minute breather from life and enjoy some downtime. Read a book, breathe, paint, color, play an instrument – it's up to you.

Get started today!

THE LIVE-IT! 180

The five **habits** you need t
order to *lose weigh*

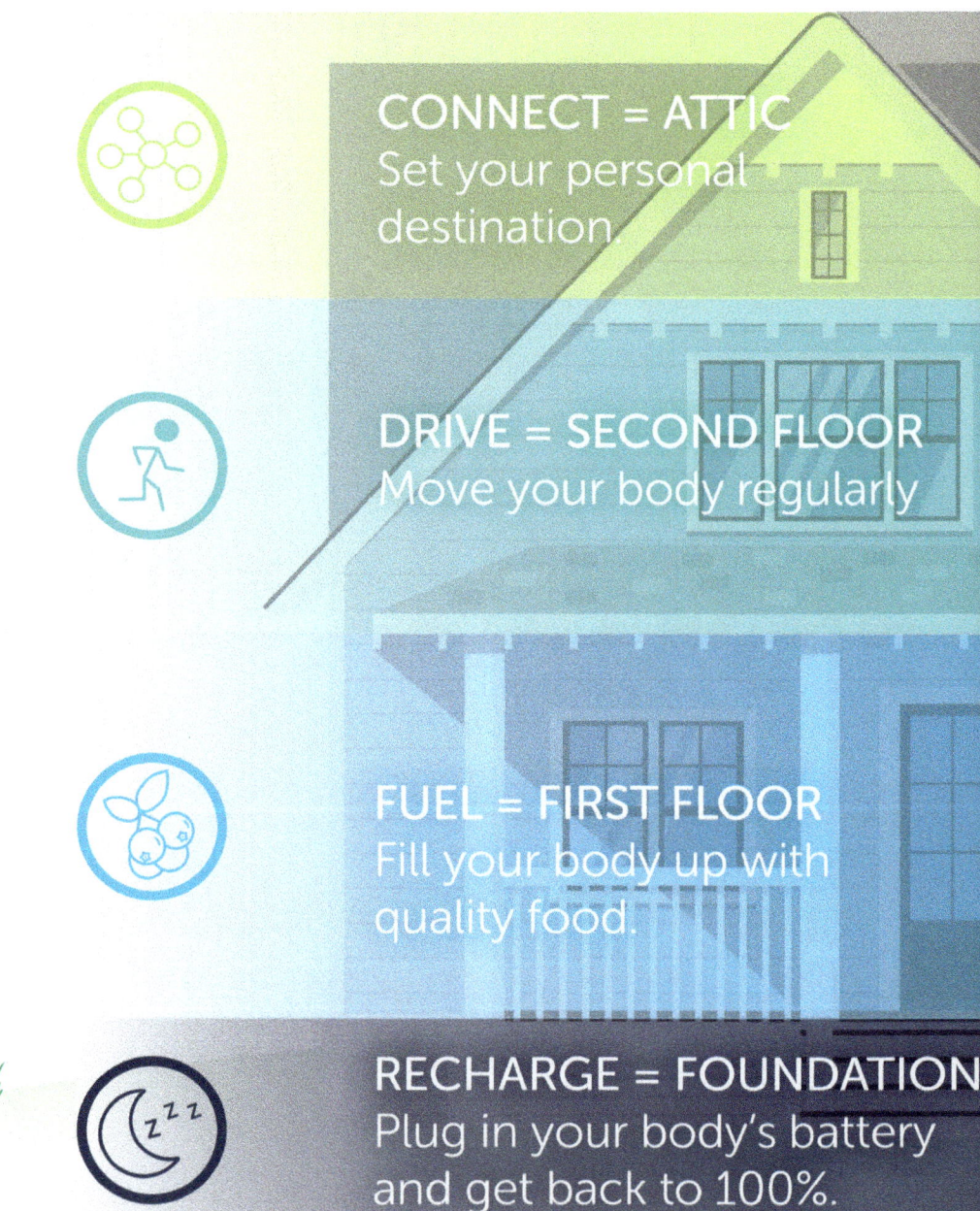

CONNECT = ATTIC
Set your personal destination.

DRIVE = SECOND FLOOR
Move your body regularly

FUEL = FIRST FLOOR
Fill your body up with quality food.

RECHARGE = FOUNDATION
Plug in your body's battery and get back to 100%.

HOUSE PLAN

build your life around in
ive fit, and *enjoy life!*

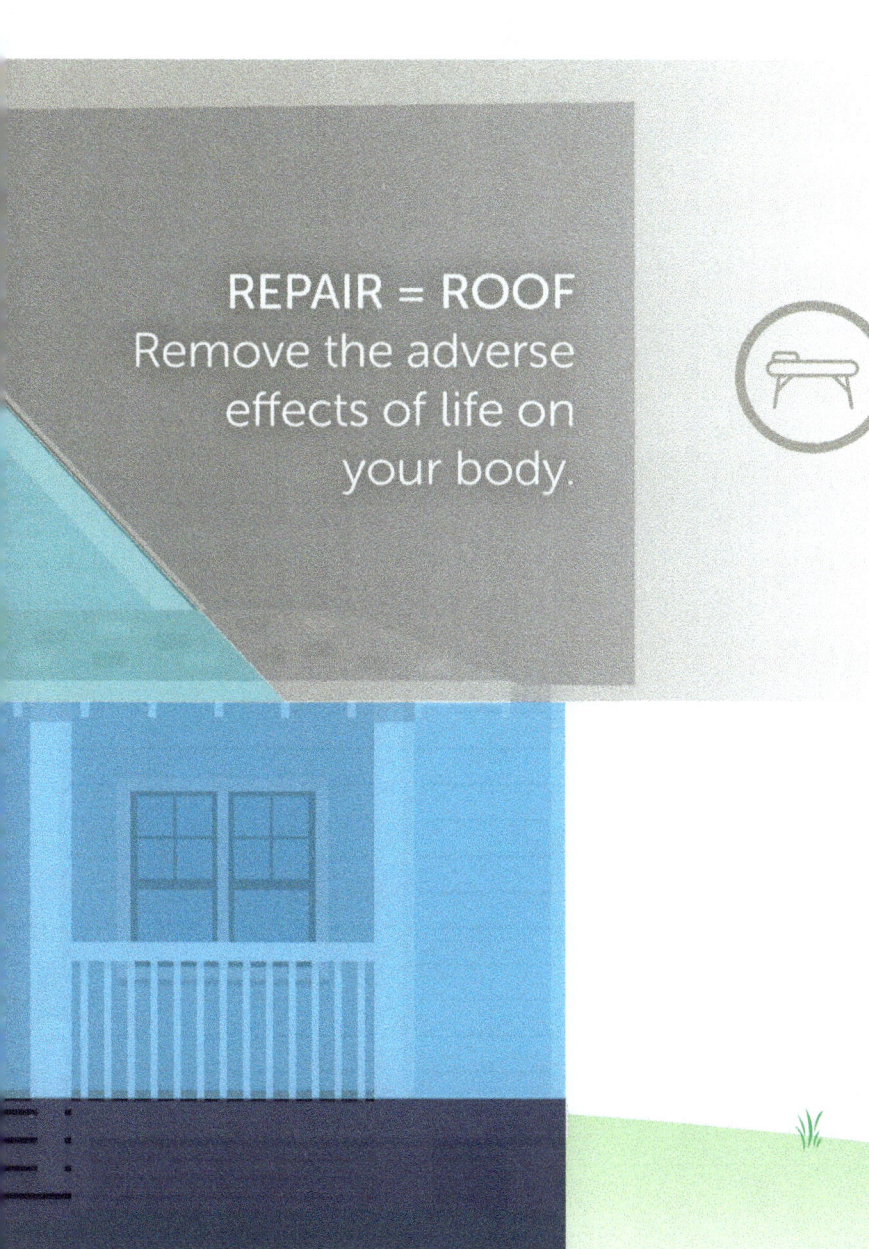

REPAIR = ROOF
Remove the adverse effects of life on your body.

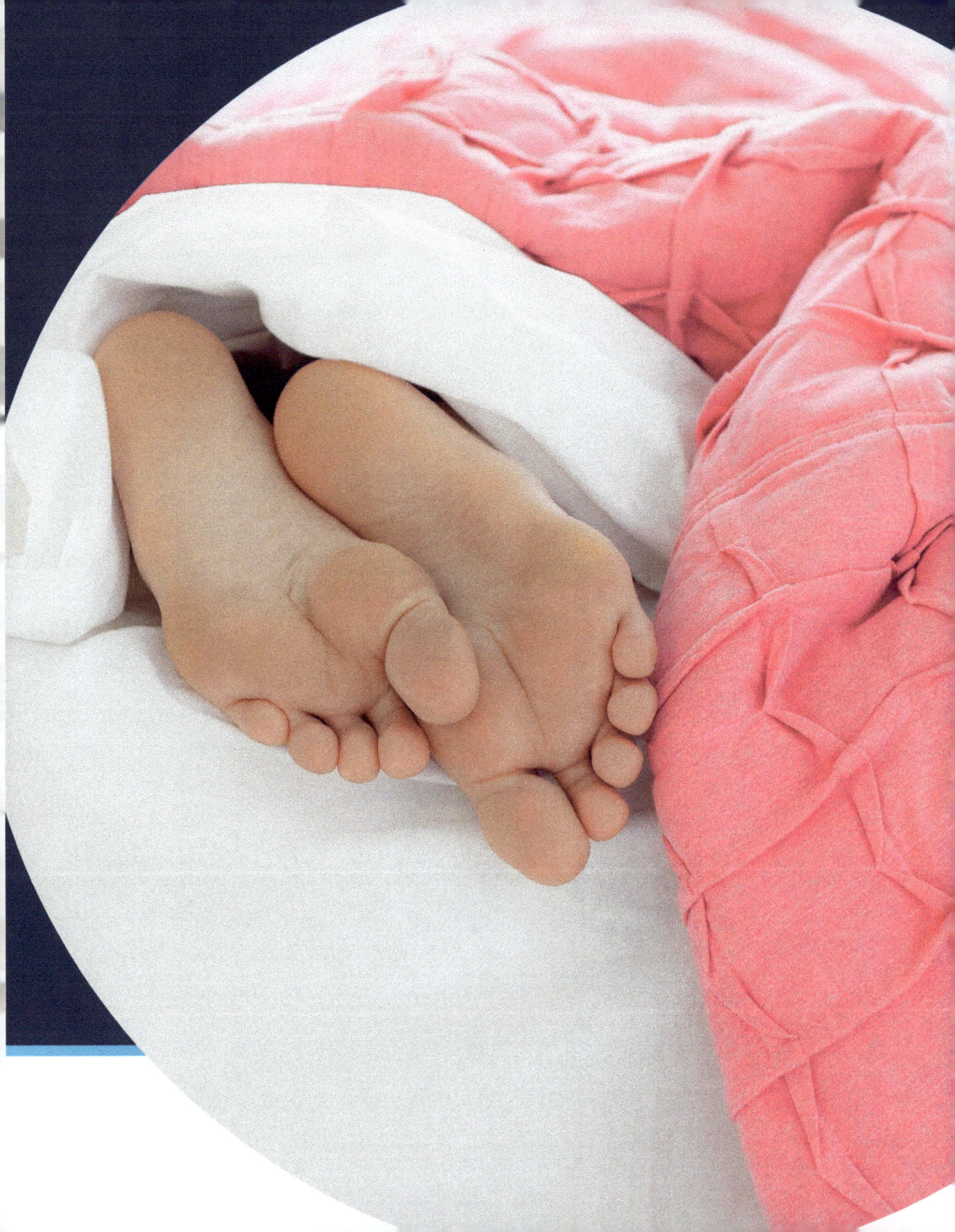

RECHARGE

Plug in your body's battery and get back to 100%.

5

You have to plug in your body's battery and get it back to 100% (by getting enough sleep)

LIVE-IT! 180° INSIGHT

If your body is an Intelligently Designed Vehicle ... and it is ... then you can think of SLEEP as the BATTERY that powers that vehicle.

When I begin to talk to people about **LIVE-IT! 180°**, they often expect me to start telling them about the importance of two things: eating and exercising. Let's face it, that's what most of us think of when we hear words like "fitness" and "health." We expect long lectures about changing what we eat and how (or whether) we exercise. Such discussions tend to make us anxious. Why? Because we've been told for so many years that what we eat and how we exercise are of massive, overwhelming importance, far outranking any other factors, when it comes to personal health. And we have a history of not doing everything we "should do" in those areas. (I know I didn't, anyway, before I had my kidney-stones episode.)

So, when I tell people that the most critical element in their personal health picture and the first principle of **LIVE-IT! 180°** is SLEEP, I get a lot of surprised looks.

Don't get me wrong. What you eat and how you move are vitally important to your health and well-being. That's why FUEL and DRIVE are the second and third principles, respectively. But the most important principle, the place where we absolutely, positively must begin, is a truly good night's sleep – which is something most of the people I talk to have not been getting.

If you aren't getting enough of the right kind of sleep, *nothing else is going to come together for you in any of the other four areas of **LIVE-IT! 180°**.*

THE BATTERY

Sleep is the driving force behind everything. It's the key component of your health and well-being ... but countless fitness "experts" de-emphasize it or overlook it entirely. Sleep is the battery that cranks everything else into action. So, sleep is what you will need to focus on as you begin to implement **LIVE-IT! 180°**.

You can skip food for a week or two without experiencing irreversible negative health effects; you can go without drinking water for perhaps two to three days without running into major trouble. Similarly, you can go for years or decades without taking part in a meaningful exercise program, and unfortunately, many people do. And yes, you can ignore your social relationships altogether and have major stress management problems, keeping up those bad habits for years or decades, progressively lowering the quality of your life, without actually dying. *But no one knows exactly how long you can survive without sleep, because the tests on humans are considered just too dangerous to conduct.*

I'm not kidding. The scientists doing the research really don't know how long you can go without sleeping before you kill yourself, and from all I can tell, they don't want to know. It's likely, though, that 72 hours of absolutely uninterrupted wakefulness constitutes a flashing red light that most people would be foolish to ignore. And even assuming that you avoid subjecting your body and your brain to that insane level of abuse, it's worth understanding the potential negative health impacts that a consistently poor night's sleep can bring about.

- An impaired immune system

- Increased risk of obesity

- Increased risk of psychiatric disorders

- Increased risk of atherosclerotic cardio-vascular (CV) disease

- Increased risk of diabetes 2

- Increased risk of impaired neurological function

- Increase risk of kidney disease

- Increased risk of suicide

> "If you aren't getting enough of the right kind of sleep, nothing else is going to come together for you in any of the other four areas of LIVE-IT! 180°."

Bad things start to happen when you try to run the Intelligently Designed machine that is your body without the battery power that drives the engine.

You can also think about your nightly sleep commitment as being similar to the battery of your cell phone. If you are getting ready for bed at eleven o'clock at night, and you notice that your cell phone charge is running low, what do you do? You plug it in, of course. Why do you plug it in? Because you know that if you don't, it's not going to do what you want in the morning. Your body works on exactly the same principle. You need to notice when your personal battery is running low and recharge it. If you don't, you're going to have trouble.

It's estimated that 30% of American adults – roughly 78 million people – consistently have difficulty getting a good night's rest. That's an epidemic. It's serious.

If you are one of the 78 million Americans mentioned above who are not getting enough

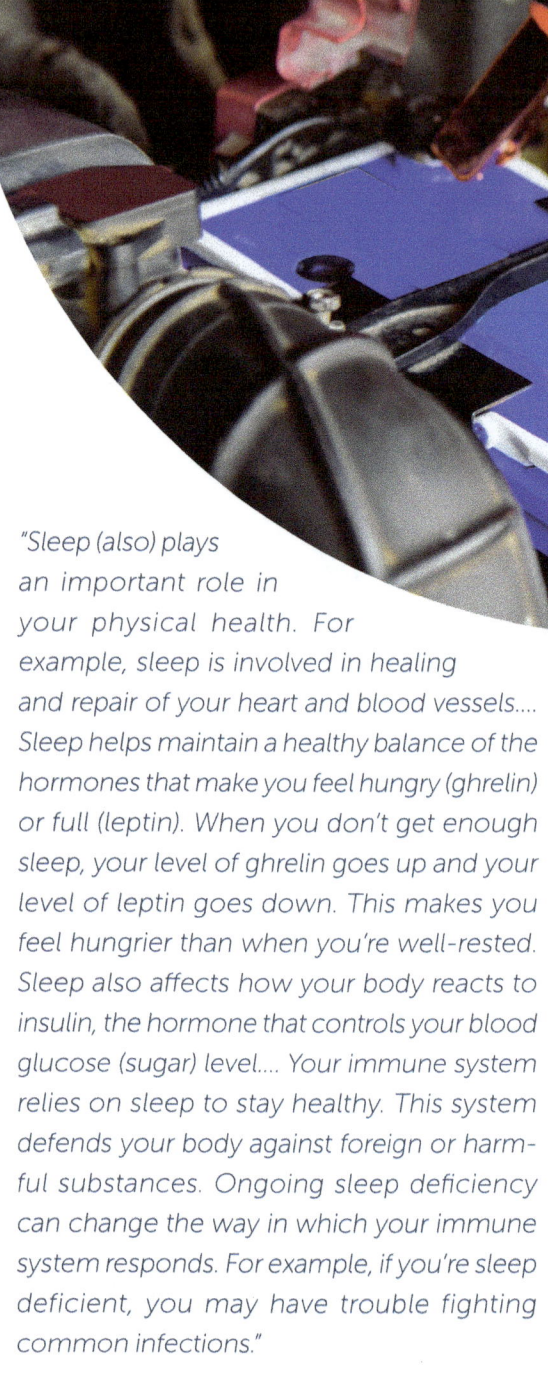

sleep, you owe it to yourself to implement the best practices that you will find in this chapter. Even if you aren't one of those people, you can use the information here to ensure you maintain healthy sleep patterns... and you can help friends and loved ones to lay a solid foundation for good personal health. Whatever you do, DO NOT SKIP THIS CHAPTER!

Consider the following powerful summary of key points from the National Institutes of Health:

> *"While you're sleeping, your brain is preparing for the next day. It's forming new pathways to help you learn and remember information. Studies show that a good night's sleep improves learning. Whether you're learning math, how to play the piano, how to perfect your golf swing, or how to drive a car, sleep helps enhance your learning and problem-solving skills. Sleep also helps you pay attention, make decisions, and be creative. If you're sleep deficient, you may have trouble making decisions, solving problems, controlling your emotions and behavior, and coping with change. Sleep deficiency also has been linked to depression, suicide, and risk-taking behavior. Children and teens who are sleep deficient may have problems getting along with others. They may feel angry and impulsive, have mood swings, feel sad or depressed, or lack motivation. They also may have problems paying attention, and they may get lower grades and feel stressed."*

> *"Sleep (also) plays an important role in your physical health. For example, sleep is involved in healing and repair of your heart and blood vessels.... Sleep helps maintain a healthy balance of the hormones that make you feel hungry (ghrelin) or full (leptin). When you don't get enough sleep, your level of ghrelin goes up and your level of leptin goes down. This makes you feel hungrier than when you're well-rested. Sleep also affects how your body reacts to insulin, the hormone that controls your blood glucose (sugar) level.... Your immune system relies on sleep to stay healthy. This system defends your body against foreign or harmful substances. Ongoing sleep deficiency can change the way in which your immune system responds. For example, if you're sleep deficient, you may have trouble fighting common infections."*

National Institutes of Health

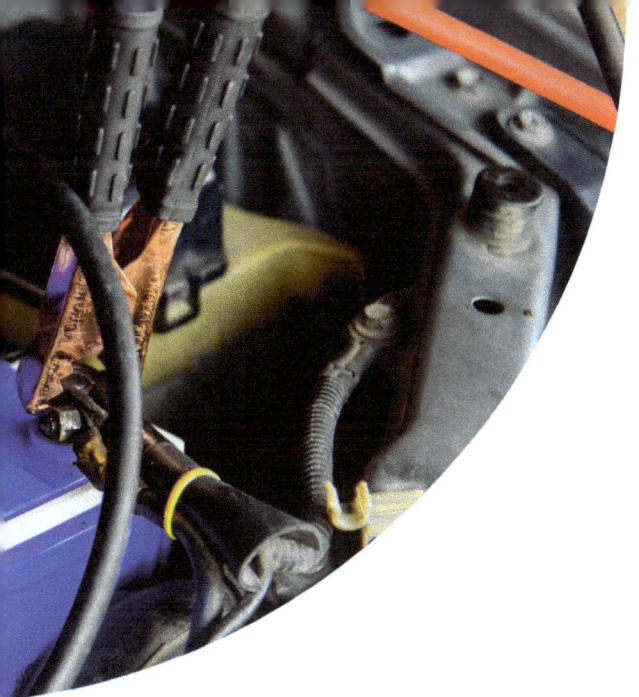

LIVE-IT! 180° INSIGHT

A good night's sleep is a "must-have," not a "nice-to-have."

WHAT HAPPENS WHEN YOU MESS UP YOUR BATTERY? (OR: HOW I TURNED MYSELF INTO A SLEEP GUINEA PIG)

To give you a sense of the kinds of strange things that can happen to your "battery" when you ignore the body's need for a good night's sleep, I want to share the results of a personal experiment I conducted recently, on myself.

Let me be clear: What I did is not something I recommend that you do or that you encourage anyone else to do. But it was enlightening.

I wanted to test the response of my own body and mind to a prolonged state of sleeplessness (I'll go into a little more detail about why I wanted to do that later). Consequently, I decided to stay up for as long as I could and keep tabs on what happened. In addition to some predictable changes – increased irritability and fatigue and decreased efficiency and detail orientation – I experienced one change that I definitely did not expect.

Before I tell you what it is, I need to make it clear to you that I'm now in very good shape physically, thanks to all the time I've spent on LIVE-IT! 180°. I do not crave sweets or sugar-laden foods. I haven't craved those kinds of foods for years now. Yet, at right about the 24-hour mark of sleeplessness, I started having an intense craving for *glazed doughnuts*.

Let me explain why this is so significant. When we shortchange ourselves on sleep, we deprive the brain of glucose, a simple sugar that's an important energy source for us. We need glucose to nourish the brain and keep ourselves alive, alert, and mobile. But when we're sleep-deprived, we start functioning with 10-15% less glucose than our brain needs. So, what happens? Well, because the brain is a critical system that has to be maintained, one of the Autopilot Conductor's self-preservation alarms goes off. In my case, it said, "Find some glazed doughnuts! Now!"

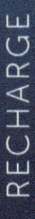

What my brain was actually saying was, "Hey, Einstein, I'm not getting the glucose I need. Take action!" Of course, extremely heavy, ongoing consumption of glucose – which is what I was longing for – carries potential negative health impacts in many other areas. (Chronically elevated blood glucose levels have been linked to decreased immunity and wound healing, nerve damage, kidney failure, obesity, heart attack, and stroke, among other problems.) But the Autopilot Conductor does what it can to preserve functioning in essential systems. The trouble is that when one system is having problems, other systems are also likely to tip into imbalance.

By the way – I did eat those glazed doughnuts. My sleep deprivation got the last word. I wonder how many poor food decisions are based on that kind of influence.

WHY I DID THIS

In case you're wondering, I kept up my sleepless stretch, under the supervision of a doctor, for ninety-four and a half hours. That's how long I was able to go before my body went into full self-preservation mode and basically ordered me to bed. Now, that's a very, very long time to go without recharging the human body's battery, and I *do not* recommend that you try this. My aim was to test exactly how long it would take my body to recover from this serious sleep deficit.

For the first few days after my sleep deficit experiment, I felt like I had been hit by a car. Even after that, my mental alertness was reduced, I lacked energy, and I had physical pain in my jaw and kidneys. It took me one week and five days to bounce back from that.

Now, most adults need seven and a half hours of sleep a night. What I figured out was that cheating my body out of the thirty hours of sleep it had coming over those four days took about two weeks of optimum performance away from me. It wasn't worth it, of course, and I hope that much is obvious to you by now.

But here's the really interesting thing: During the last three days of my recovery from the experiment, I remembered that years before, when I wasn't taking care of myself and wasn't making sure I got my seven and a half hours sleep a night, I had *felt that way most of the time*. Poor sleep patterns were part of the reason my car was headed for the cliff.

I remembered that sluggishness. I remembered that difficulty getting things started in the morning. I remembered the short attention span. I remembered the even shorter temper. I remembered the sensation (usually accurate) that I had overlooked something important.

I realized that I used to live my life in a constant state of recovery and a perpetually unpaid sleep debt. It wasn't a good way to live.

It may have been reckless for me to go nearly four days without sleep – but it was just as reckless, years ago, for me to put myself in a constant state of sleep debt. At least this time around, I knew I was making a mistake – and I caught up!

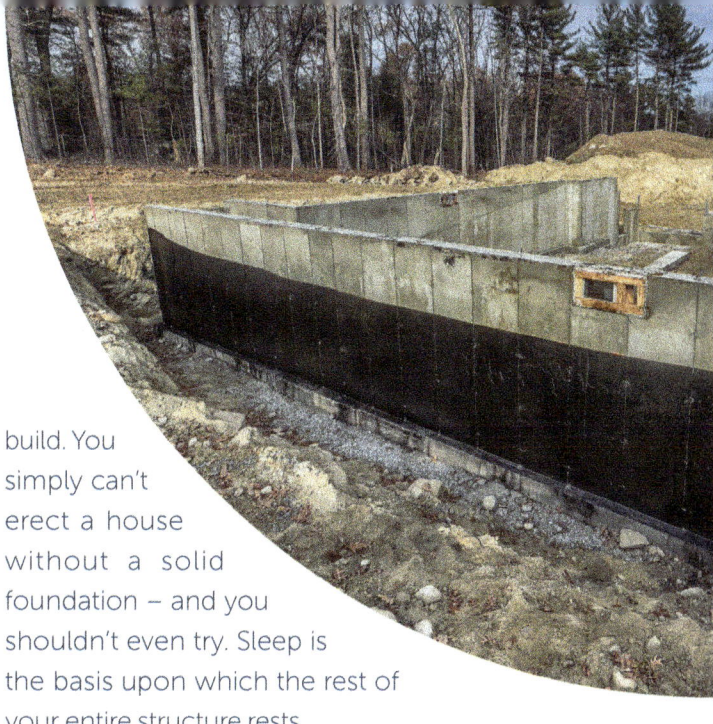

Your Intelligently Designed body allows you to miss sleep you need ... and still function ... but you have to catch up. You have to pay the debt back. Interestingly, there is no way to build up a "surplus" in your sleep bank. All you can do is bring a negative balance back up to zero. Failing to do that leaves you in a state of chronic fatigue that not only carries all kinds of adverse health impacts, but also makes it impossible for you to benefit from LIVE-IT! 180°.

build. You simply can't erect a house without a solid foundation – and you shouldn't even try. Sleep is the basis upon which the rest of your entire structure rests.

If you have that foundation in place, you'll have the solid footing you need to make steady progress with the other four LIVE-IT! 180° principles. On the other hand, if you don't have the foundation in place, nothing else will stand up!

Everything will sink if the foundation isn't sound. If your house is tipping into the abyss due to a bad foundation, none of the carpentry will matter, none of the electrical work or the plumbing will matter, and none of the finish work will matter.

Each of the five LIVE-IT! 180° principles is interconnected with the other four, but *nothing* good can happen in terms of your progress on principles Two through Five until you've laid down a solid foundation with principle One: Recharge. That's how important your sleep patterns are.

LIVE-IT! 180° INSIGHT

The moral: If you are perpetually overdrawn at the sleep bank, you are setting yourself up for disaster. Don't tell yourself this is normal. It's not!

THE FOUNDATION

As you move forward with LIVE-IT! 180°, I want to challenge you to think of your sleep pattern as being like the foundation of a house you want to

RECHARGE

CHALLENGE THE STATUS QUO

Making positive changes in our life only happens when we create meaningful habits... and changing our habits only happens when we find powerful *reasons* to change. So, what are some good reasons to change your habits and ensure you get a better night's sleep?

Consider the following list closely – and *share it with a partner.*

Top 10 Reasons to Change Your SLEEP Status Quo

10. *Inadequate sleep makes you ugly.* That's not exactly a scientific finding, because physical attractiveness is a subjective thing, but it is an important factor, and if you think back on what your own experience is with missing out on sleep and what you see when you check the mirror the next morning, you'll realize that this is a real issue. Come on, put down the makeup or the denial, whichever you're more likely to use next. Pay attention to this. You know it's true. Cutting corners on your sleep at night makes you less attractive the next day. In and of itself, that's enough of a reason to challenge the status quo.

9. *Inadequate sleep makes you irritable, angry, hostile, and depressed.* This one *is scientifically* verifiable (See "*Up All Night: The Effects of Sleep Loss on Mood*," in Psychology Today, August 13, 2015 - bit.ly/liveit1). If you've experienced any or all of these states and assumed they came about due to your surroundings, your bad luck, or the people around you, you owe it to yourself and your loved ones to change what you're doing in terms of your sleep patterns.

8. *Inadequate sleep adversely affects your hormone levels.* There is an intricate dance your body does to keep the right hormones coursing through your body at the right time of day, and getting enough sleep is a critical element of that dance. Messing up the sleep dance makes the mood problems I mentioned in #9 above much more likely. Not only that: When you don't get enough sleep, you restrict the time available to your body for the release of the hormones essential for growing and repairing muscles and reducing belly fat.

7. *Inadequate sleep causes all kinds of complex negative internal stresses.* A classic example of this is our body's production of the hormone known as cortisol. This naturally occurring hormone is meant to get us up in the morning. When we mess up our own sleep patterns, however, we tend to overload on cortisol to get through the day. If this happens regularly, it carries all kinds of problems. Our cortisol level is supposed to dip down at nighttime, allowing us to feel calmer and recharge. When cortisol levels are too high – something that can be caused by stress as well as lack of sleep – we may notice that we get a "second wind" around bedtime, even though we've been tired all day long. This is not good. Why not? Because even though we're exhausted, we toss and turn all night, thereby starting the cycle all over again, only worse. (By the way, I believe that an internal overload of cortisol is the #1 reason we have too much belly fat.)

6. Inadequate sleep makes it hard, and sometimes impossible, for you to make good choices in other areas of your life. Remember those glazed doughnuts I ate? Bad choices tend to cascade and build off one another, creating an accelerating "tsunami effect" of increasingly terrible decisions in terms of the food you eat, your physical activity, the quality of your relationships, and the way you manage stress (or don't). The bad decision cycle usually starts with the core bad habit a lot of us have of short-changing ourselves when it comes to getting a good night's sleep. We need to change that habit!

5. Inadequate sleep messes up your brain's ability to function. I don't know about you, but I'm not keen on degrading my brainpower. When the body is asleep and resting, there is time for fluids to flush in and out of the brain. This process is another part of Intelligent Design that's worth understanding. Discover more about how your brain uses sleep to wash itself free of toxins at http://bit.ly/liveit2. This cerebrospinal fluid wash is like cleaning up the hard drive on your computer with CleanDisk or a similar application. It removes bad stuff, fragments, and any number of extra bits that aren't needed, and sets up better pathways, so the brain operates faster and more effectively. But you don't have to buy, activate, or launch a piece of software to get this to happen. All you have to do is get a good night's sleep.

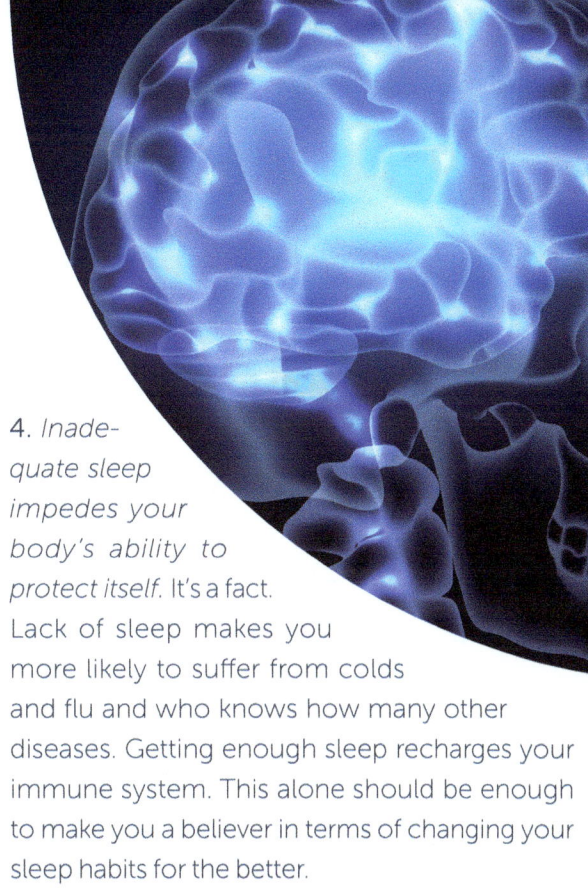

4. Inadequate sleep impedes your body's ability to protect itself. It's a fact. Lack of sleep makes you more likely to suffer from colds and flu and who knows how many other diseases. Getting enough sleep recharges your immune system. This alone should be enough to make you a believer in terms of changing your sleep habits for the better.

3. For many people, inadequate sleep is linked to blood sugar problems. This is a big deal. Over time, blood sugar problems are known to contribute to diabetes, heart disease, and cancer.

2. Inadequate sleep affects learning and memory. Your ability to focus and learn efficiently are directly correlated to the quality of your sleep. When you get a lousy night's sleep, memories don't "stick" the way they should. It's that simple.

1. Inadequate sleep can cause problems in your sex life. Poor sleep patterns lower libido levels for both genders and make some men significantly less likely to have and maintain an erection. If that's not an argument in favor of changing the status

RECHARGE

67

quo, I don't know what is! (By the way, we'll cover libido issues and other important health challenges you may face in the OBSTACLES chapter of this book.)

THE BOTTOM LINE: If you don't do everything necessary to get between seven-and-a-half and nine hours of sleep tonight, you will be VOLUNTEERING to run into ALL TEN of the big problems you just read about – and you will probably run into them sooner rather than later. To keep that from happening ... read on!

> " These cycles need to unfold uninterrupted in order for us to get the rest we need."

THE BASICS: WHAT YOU NEED TO KNOW ABOUT YOUR SLEEP PATTERN

It's not just a question of the amount of sleep you get – the quality *of sleep you get is equally important.*

The human sleep cycle, a natural miracle that restores and heals us, is a core component of our Intelligent Design. That cycle plays out in roughly 90-minute cycles. Each 90-minute cycle needs to cover four stages in order to protect, heal, and restore our bodies and minds. Those four cycles are:

STAGE ONE. This is the transition between wakefulness and sleep. It's where we begin to relax our muscles and notice that we are having difficulty keeping our eyes open. We are still aware of our surroundings.

STAGE TWO: We become less aware of our surroundings. Our body temperature drops. Our breathing and heart rate become more regular. Our muscles relax further.

STAGE THREE: Our muscles continue to relax, our blood pressure and breathing rates drop, and we are no longer aware of our surroundings at all.

STAGE FOUR: We experience rapid eye movement (REM) sleep, which is marked by vivid dreams and high brain activity. Our body, which is relaxed and immobile, turns inward and pays attention to internal messages.

When all this happens within a 90-minute cycle, we benefit. Our body and mind can start to repair itself from all the stresses of the day, and our system can start to come back into balance. It's really a miracle!

PUTTING IT ALL TOGETHER

To get an ideal night's rest, we need to string a number of those cycles together. As it turns out, that's exactly how we're designed. At the end of the first cycle, the process starts all over again, skipping the first transition phase and returning to Stage Two. Depending on our body's requirements, we may experience a total of five or six of these ninety-minute cycles during the course of a good night's sleep.

The point to remember is, these cycles need to unfold *uninterrupted* in order for us to get the rest we need. For that to happen, there are certain "non-negotiables" our body demands from us. In order for you to get a good night's sleep, you must:

- **Set aside a specific time that you plan to go to bed and a specific time you plan to get up, and make sure that the span of time you set aside equals *at least* seven and a half hours.** You can allow up to nine hours if you want, but it must be at least seven and a half. *If there's no plan, you're not going to get the result you want.* So, make the plan and stick to it. (Yes, this includes Fridays and weekends.)

- **Give yourself a "cool-down" period of at least 30 minutes *before* the time you've established you will go to bed.** If you plan to go to bed at 10 pm, make sure your "cool-down" period begins by 9:30. What makes this period of time different from the rest of the day? Simple. No food or drink. No TV. No phones. No Internet. No videogames. In short, nothing you have to digest and nothing with a screen. Now, before you get too busy focusing on what you *can't* do during this period, let me share a list of things you *can* do during the "cool-down" period. You can read a book – the old-fashioned kind with pages that you turn. You can organize your thoughts for the next day by making a list of things you want to do. You can get out your breakfast prep (you'll be learning more about that in the next chapter) and lay out your clothes. You can meditate. If you have a sauna or jacuzzi, you can use that. You can also relax in any way you see fit with your spouse or significant other. Hey, your relationship just got better.

- **When you go to bed, turn off all the lights and close all the curtains.** Make sure the room is completely dark when you start your first sleep cycle.

Do these three non-negotiables always come easily to people who are used to the relentless, unforgiving, punishing pace of 21st-century media addiction? No.

Are they still non-negotiable, both for you and your accountability partner, as you each create

RECHARGE

69

your personal **LIVE-IT! 180°** lifestyle? Yes.

Of course, I realize the world we live in often seems to be designed to tempt you to break all three of these commitments – and let's face it, that's probably what you're used to doing. It's what I was used to doing. I didn't plan my sleep pattern. I went pedal to the metal, full throttle, 100% intensity all the way, snacking and drinking soda until I got to the point where I realized I was exhausted and I thought, "OK, time to go to bed." Then I flipped on the TV and stared into the electric void until I conked out.

The problem with that approach is that it robbed me of almost all the benefits of a good night's sleep.

Think about it. If I'm supposed to get up at six and I don't fall asleep until one AM, I lose out on at least the first of the five 90-minute sleep cycles I need. That's not good.

Even worse, by snacking and drinking during what should have been my cool-down period, I made my body work to digest the food at a time when it needed to use that energy to get my brain into the first restful, repairing, miraculous phase of REM sleep. Once again, I missed out. Of course, if I had to get up in the middle of the night to pee, which I often did, I made the problem even worse.

And guess what? By leaving the TV and other lights on long into the night, I was severely degrading my body's ability to get me into that REM phase.

CIRCADIAN RHYTHM: What does that mean?

Your circadian rhythm is a cycle of roughly 24 hours that tells your body when to sleep, when to wake up, and when to eat. The word "circadian" comes from a Latin phrase meaning "around one day." This rhythm controls many physiological processes and serves as an internal body clock. Studies have shown that it is affected by environmental signals, like sunlight and temperature.

All too often, I never got there. As a result, I would wake up restless, exhausted, out of balance, and increasingly addicted to my own cortisol. My circadian rhythms were in a state of barely contained chaos. I was a disaster waiting to happen, a walking zombie in a state of chronic sleep debt.

Now, if my experiences sound familiar to you, and I bet they do, that's good. I want you to use that sense of dawning awareness that's creeping over you right now, and I want you to reach out to your accountability partner. Make the commitment, right out loud, to give your body the sleep it needs. Make the commitment to follow the three **LIVE-IT! 180°** non-negotiables for a good night's sleep. Ask your accountability partner to do the same. Then move on to the next phase of planning.

GOOD, BETTER, **BEST**: PERSONALIZE LIVE-IT! 180°!

Not everyone will approach this first principle of **LIVE-IT! 180°** in the same way or with the same degree of discipline. As you will see, there are multiple ways to do this "right." Here's how it breaks down.

"GOOD" – PHASE ONE

- Commit to, and follow through on, the three non-negotiables of a good night's sleep.

- Don't eat within 90 minutes before the time you go to sleep. However, you do want to make sure you *have* eaten dinner or your evening meal (something substantial and healthy) before that point. If you are planning to get to sleep at 10:00, make sure all eating is done by 8:30. Your body needs the energy from that food to run its complete heal-and-restore process on your body and mind when you go to sleep, but it also needs at least 90 minutes before you sleep to break the food down.

- Set an alarm clock to wake you up at the time you choose. (You may eventually outgrow the need for this, but for now, use the alarm clock for at least two weeks to establish a routine your body can learn to recognize... and to guarantee that you are getting at least seven and a half hours of sleep.)

You can stop there or move on to...

"BETTER" – PHASE TWO

Do everything in the "GOOD" phase and add the following steps:

- Use lavender and/or peppermint extracts, sprinkled on a hot damp washcloth, to help you relax during your cool-down period. Spread the washcloth over your face and breathe slow and deep for a few minutes. Aaaah.

- Take a shower or bath during your cool-down period to release the day's stress, cleanse the body, and prepare for rest. Decompress.

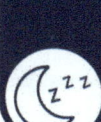

"BEST" – PHASE THREE

Do everything in the "GOOD" and "BETTER" phases and add the following steps:

- Redesign your sleep space completely. Reclaim it. To start with, make sure the room in which you sleep is totally sealed off and *pitch dark* when it's time to go to sleep. That means no moonlight. No electric light. No street light. Nothing! Turn this space into your "sleep cave." Don't allow electronics into this room – ever. In fact, don't do *anything* in this room except for cooling down, reading, intimacy with your partner, and sleep. Make it a sacred space – and keep it sacred!

A FINAL THOUGHT

Will emergencies happen from time to time? Will a big storm hit? Will one of your kids have a nightmare and need consoling? Will there be other good reasons to get up at 2:00 AM and deal with reality?

Of course. But that's no reason not to set and reinforce a sleep routine.

The key word there is "routine." What matters, when it comes to sleep, is what you can turn into a habit that your body learns to predict and expect. *Your body needs this routine.* Don't get distracted by what only happens occasionally. Plan for what usually happens – and make sure it supports you.

> "Even a soul submerged in sleep is hard at work and helps make something of the world."
> —Heraclitus

Plan your life and live your plan. LIVE-IT! 180°.

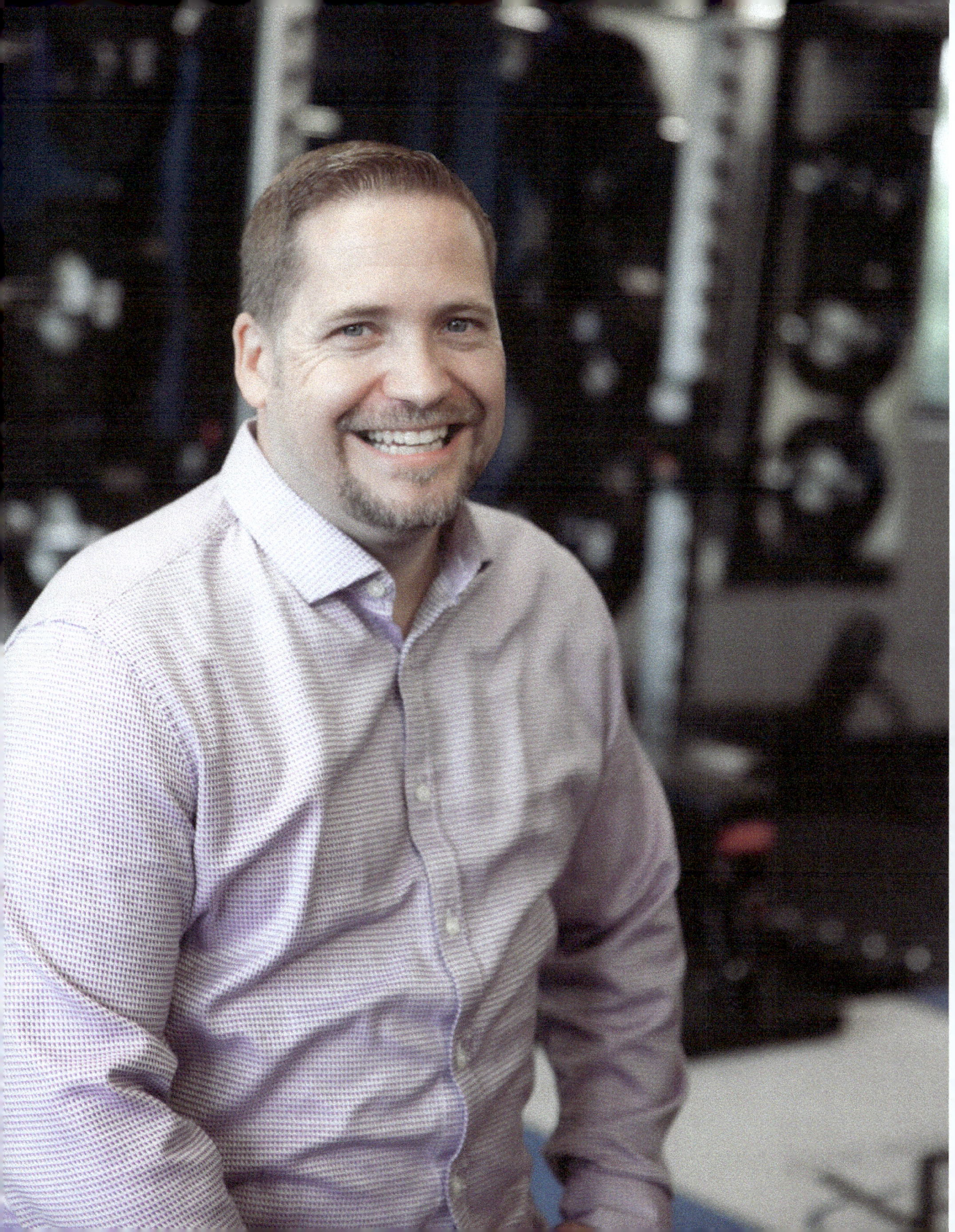

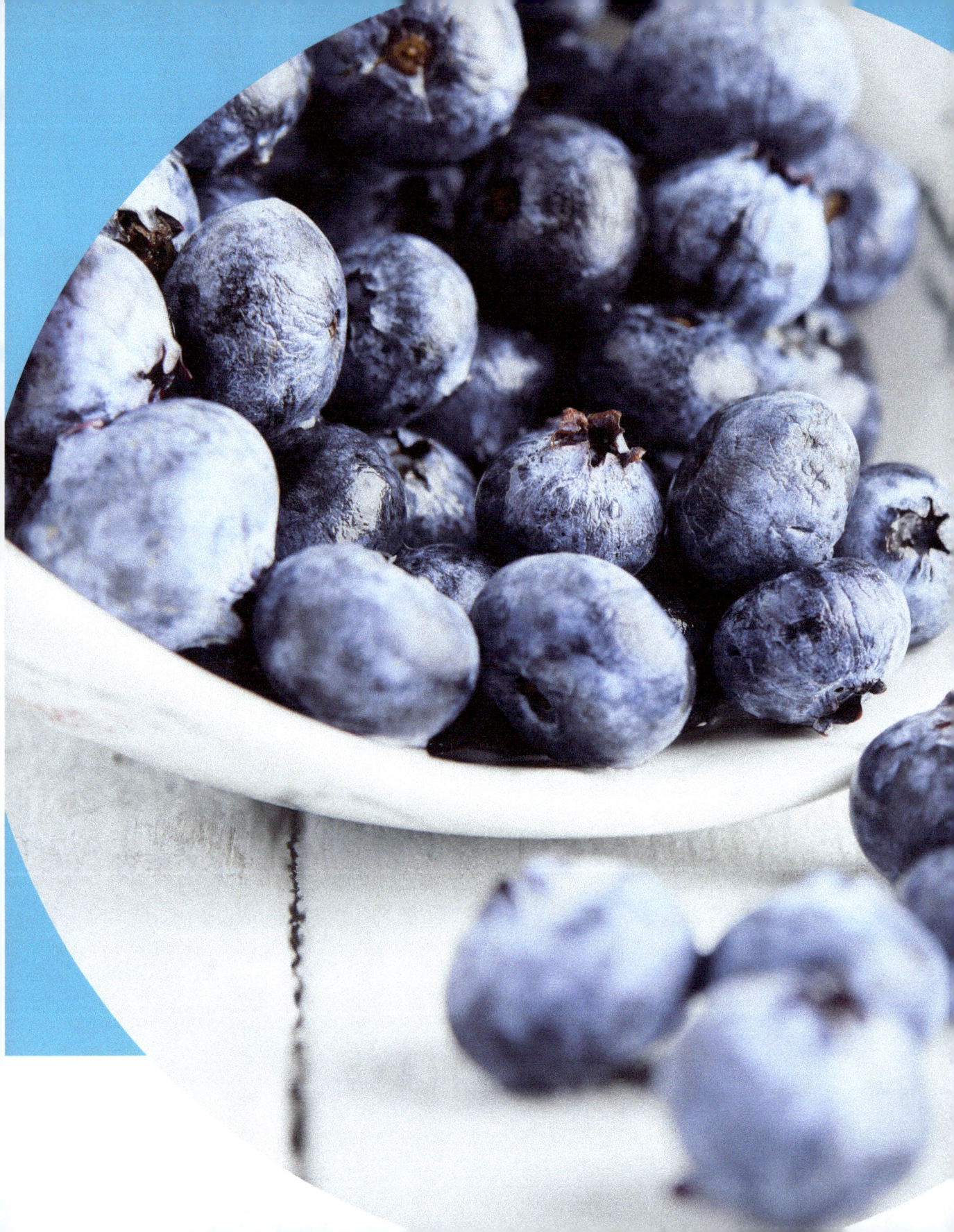

FUEL

Fill your body up with quality food by eating right according to your body design.

6

You have to fill up your body with quality food (by eating right)

In the previous chapter, I asked you to think of sleep as the battery that starts your car. Now, I want you to think of food as the FUEL that powers that Intelligently Designed car.

Bear in mind that this is a sophisticated vehicle, a supercar. You can choose to put high-octane fuel in it, as the manufacturer recommends, or you can choose to put cheap fuel in it. Your choices will affect the vehicle's performance.

THE BIG ONE

As you know, all the **LIVE-IT! 180°** principles are important, all of them are interconnected, and all of them require the kind of commitment that comes only with a personalized routine, one that you discuss regularly with your accountability partner. I've found, however, that there's something special about our relationship with the food we eat, something that makes fulfilling this second principle a special challenge. For many of us, what we eat is "the big one," the issue we have a lot of emotion around and maybe a lot of experience in trying to change.

So, I'm going to spend a lot of time on this principle to make sure that you and your accountability partner get all the resources and information you need to execute it properly and to support yourselves as you move through the system. I ask that you spend as much time as necessary on this chapter, too.

BEYOND "GOING ON A DIET"

Let's begin at the beginning. Too many of us have been trained to think of "good health" as being synonymous with this elaborate, painful, complex process called "going on a diet." Too many of us have bought into that myth, come up short, failed to get the results we wanted, and assumed that the problem was something we did. We didn't pick the "right" diet (and of course there are dozens to choose from), or we didn't follow the diet properly, or we didn't go to the right support group, or we didn't buy the right "diet" soda, or whatever.

It's all a bunch of lies.

The problem wasn't anything we did. The problem is that there are multi-billion-dollar industries based on getting us to assume, among other things, that adjusting what we eat is the key to perfect health. These industries are supported by powerful industrial and governmental interests. In other words, it's in certain elite interests for us to oversimplify, buy food that isn't as wholesome and nutritious as it needs to be, make bad eating choices, and bounce from diet to diet.

But it's not in our interest to do that. And we don't have to.

LIVE-IT! 180° addresses not only diet, but our lives as a whole. The body is far too complex to minimize all the relevant issues down to just food. The real problem is the "experts" who take a limited, short-sighted approach to human health and the industries that shove "ghost food" into our cupboards and refrigerators, onto our dinner plates, and down our throats.

In a world where advertisements, government agencies, and social media all tell us the type of food to eat (and, all too often, point us toward overprocessed "ghost food" that has been stripped of most essential nutrients), it's no wonder that so many people in our society are fat, unhappy, and living simply to die. That outcome is a function of the world that has been built around us.

We live in a world that ridicules you if you want to be healthy, eat organic, live responsibly, and ignore mainstream brainwashing in order to achieve wellness and regain control of your life. We live in a world that wants you to believe it's a complex and difficult task to make food choices that help you to live how you were designed to live. We live in a world that goes out of its way to make changing how you eat inconvenient and unpopular.

The good news is, we can change all that. If we choose to change it.

The first step to change is knowledge. We have to ask ourselves, "Why is it so hard for so many people in our society to change their eating patterns?" The answer lies in one simple word: greed.

"We can change all that. If we choose to change it."

Big business (both the huge diet industry and the various arms of the even larger food industry) pumps a ton of money into advertising, deception, and flawed studies to convince us that certain foods and certain dietary approaches are good for us or, at best, won't hurt us. They often lie. The government, on the whole, is okay with that. It does not protect consumers and does not stand up for the less fortunate and less informed in our society, who have blindly placed trust in the government to protect their interests over those of big business.

In this chapter, I'm going to share with you how powerful interests have rigged the game, why you shouldn't let them, and what you can do instead when it comes to choosing what you eat.

WHAT BIG FOOD DOESN'T WANT YOU TO KNOW

Let's start with something important, something that the complex industrial and governmental alliances that I'll call Big Food would rather you didn't know. If you buy your food through the stores and restaurants most people buy from, the food you eat today is fundamentally different from the food most people in America ate in the first half of the twentieth century. And when I say "fundamen-

tally different," I don't mean at the level of spice or presentation. I mean the food is *chemically different* and *nutritionally inferior* to what people ate in the past.

If you were feeling hungry, how would you feel if I offered you a plastic garbage can lid with some Vaseline spread across the top of it and said, "Bon appetit?"

You'd probably think I was insane. And you know what? You'd be right. But that's basically what you're leaving yourself open to every time you eat something with an ingredient listing that includes "artificial flavor" – which makes up a huge percentage of the food consumed by the average American.

So, here's the truth Big Food would rather I not talk about. Every time you see the words "artificial flavor" in an ingredient list, which is disturbingly often, and you decide to eat the food anyway, you're exposing your body to at least one of about five hundred strange chemical cocktails, encompassing over two thousand different chemicals, some of which – maybe all of which – are linked to substances you absolutely, positively would never consciously choose to eat. Like plastic (which is why I mentioned the garbage can lid). And petroleum (which is why I mentioned Vaseline).

And it's all legal. Big Food has set the system up in such a way that, under current law, it doesn't have to tell you when it puts strange stuff into the food it wants you to eat. They don't have to break down

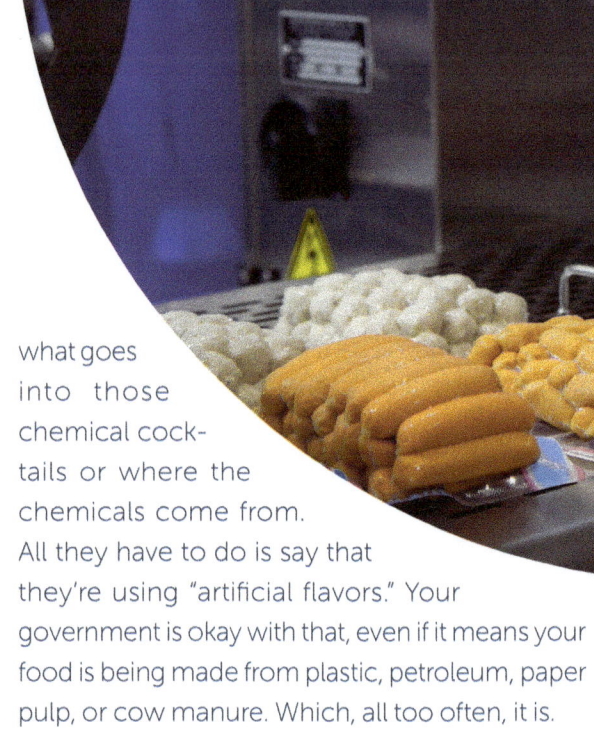

what goes into those chemical cocktails or where the chemicals come from. All they have to do is say that they're using "artificial flavors." Your government is okay with that, even if it means your food is being made from plastic, petroleum, paper pulp, or cow manure. Which, all too often, it is.

Your government has let you down. You must look out for your own interests when it comes to the food you put into your body.

I don't know about you, but when someone puts gasoline, plastic, or other dubious stuff into my food, I want to know about it ahead of time, so I can avoid eating it. I want a warning label. But our government doesn't see fit to regulate Big Food like that. As a result, *much of what Big Food channels into the world's food supply degrades the nutritional value of the food in question and/or makes it harmful.* In order to complete the FUEL principle of **LIVE-IT! 180°**, you will need to start leaning away from food that's been messed with and start leaning toward food that's hasn't, like the food people ate a century or so ago.

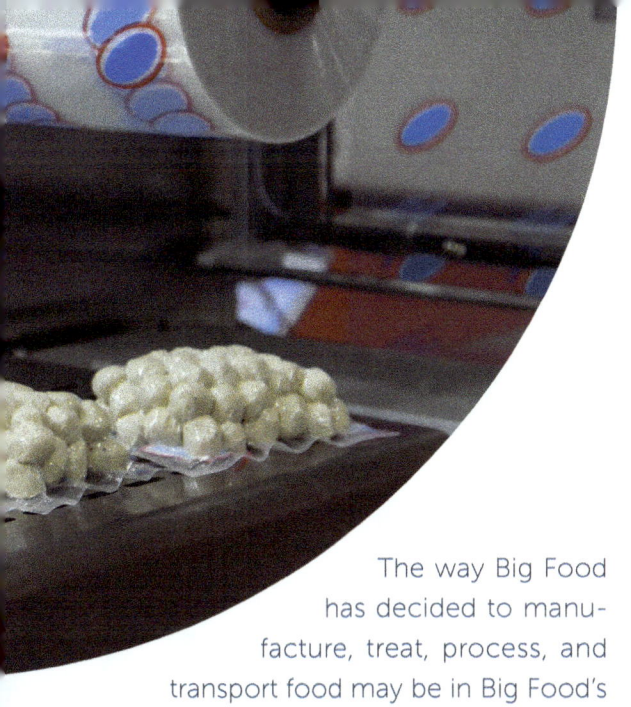

LIVE-IT! 180° INSIGHT

Big Food increases its profits by selling you chemically compromised "ghost food," designed first and foremost for mass production and distribution, which needlessly taxes your immune system and cheats you of the nutrients your body needs. You don't have to eat that food.

The way Big Food has decided to manufacture, treat, process, and transport food may be in Big Food's economic interests, but it's definitely not in your body's best interest!

Why does Big Food do this? Simple. To cut costs. To make it a little less expensive for that bag of chips or that package of frozen macaroni and cheese or that instant soup mix to make it out of the factory, onto the supermarket shelf, into your shopping card, onto your plate, and into your body. Making the food a little less expensive to produce makes it more profitable when sold. And that's good for Big Food. **But what's good for Big Food is not – I repeat –** *is not* **good for you.**

Here's the bottom line. Unless you're growing it in your backyard or getting it from a farmer's market or some other trusted source, your default position should be to assume that the food in question is compromised. Your starting position should be that you refuse to compromise when it comes to the quality of the fuel you put into the Intelligently Designed machine that is your body.

LIVE-IT! 180°'s EAT principle makes finding quality food simple and easy.

This will mean some changes in habit, but those changes are worth it. And **LIVE-IT! 180°** will help you to make them.

Not changing your habits means continuing to rely on the "ghost food" that turns a profit for Big Food and throws junk into your fuel tank. That's not what you want to do.

I'll be returning to the topic of Big Food's profit-driven compromises, and how those compromises affect your body, later in this chapter. Right now, though, I want to share some important insights into how your body processes the fuel you give it. It's a complex topic, but I think we can make it a little more straightforward with a couple of metaphors.

FUEL

79

> "Only approved macro and micro nutrients are allowed to pass."

The Straw or Barrier Wall

I want you to think of everything that happens to food as it travels between your mouth and your bum as passing through a straw – a barrier wall. I want you to consider the possibility that the act of chewing something and swallowing it doesn't actually put it "into" your body.

The stuff we eat enters our mouths, passes through our stomachs, enters the small and large intestines, and comes out the other end without ever being "inside" our bodies. In fact, all foods and liquids remain essentially "outside" our bodies until they are absorbed through our digestive tract.

This analogy is an important one: There is a barrier between the outside world and our internal world and only approved macro and micro nutrients are allowed to get in. Just like a straw placed inside a glass of water separates the water inside the straw from the rest of the water in the glass, the nutrients in our food are kept separate from the systems that need those nutrients until they have been filtered through the digestive system.

If you're having trouble with the biology here, just remember: Water doesn't go through the walls of the straw, it needs to be drawn in. Got it?

The Nightclub

You're probably wondering *how* the nutrients get from inside the straw (that is, from your mouth to your bum) and into the rest of the body (via your digestive tract.) Here's how.

Picture a big nightclub that's really popular. There are bouncers out front. The bouncers' job is to keep people out of the club who don't belong. The bouncers won't let you in if the club is too full or if you aren't wearing the right clothes, aren't on the approved list, or haven't paid your admission. If you're shrewd enough to fool the bouncers – by dressing right, for instance, or pretending to be on the appropriate list – you might be able to fake your way into the club. Once you get inside, though, and it's discovered that you don't really belong there, what's going to happen? The nightclub's security people will search the club for you, so they can grab you and throw you out.

In this particular nightclub, you look like lots of people who do belong there. As a result, when the security people search for you, they throw out many other people who were on the list, people who ought to be allowed to stay in the club. At this very security-conscious nightclub, it's not just people who don't really belong in the club

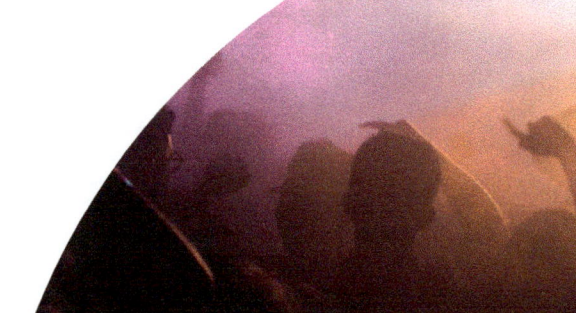

who find themselves out on the street. It's people who are on the VIP list who happen to resemble the ones who crashed the party.

That analogy explains what happens with our immune system. The walls of

our intestines block stuff from coming into the body that the body doesn't need. So, it keeps that stuff in the straw or behind the barrier wall. Unfortunately, Big Food has created new kinds of "empty food" – food that knows how to get past the bouncers, food that looks like the stuff your body needs, smells like the stuff your body needs ... but *isn't*. This "empty food" or "ghost food" goes into the body, gets past the bouncers, and it then goes into hiding. Before long, the alarms go off, and when they do, the security guards, your immune system, go looking for the intruders so they can throw them out.

Here's the good news: Your immune system can grab all this junk hiding in your cells. Here's the bad news: At the same time, your immune system robs your body of critical macronutrients, because this masked, fake food is made to look like real **macronutrients** needed by the body. Your antibodies, as they're searching out the bad stuff, actually destroy the good stuff, too.

"MACRONUTRIENTS": What does that mean?

A macronutrient is a nutrient required in large quantities every day by your Intelligently Designed body. Most dietitians identify three macronutrients: **proteins**, which are essential for the growth and repair of body tissues; **carbohydrates**, your body's go-to fuel source, and **fats**, also known as lipids, which are composed of various types of fatty acid. A word or two is in order about that last item. You do need a certain amount of fat in your daily intake, but it's important to make sure it's the right kind of fat, in the right quantity. **LIVE-IT! 180°** makes it easy for you to get the right amount of all three macronutrients into your system each day.

The problem is that your body needs these macronutrients – proteins, carbohydrates, fats – and the process that destroys the good stuff along with the bad stuff makes it harder for your body to get them. This leads to deficiencies, an overactive immune system, and systemic inflammation, which in turn, leads to aches and pains, chronic conditions such as Crohn's, and eventually disease and system failure.

81

Here's one big takeaway: This destroying-the-good-stuff cycle can intensify, depending on how much of Big Food's compromised "ghost food" we throw into our system.

Here's another big takeaway: What's going down the straw or getting past the security guards into the "nightclub" better be the good stuff, because if it isn't, alarms will go off ... and we're going to run the risk of some serious health problems.

MOVING BEYOND GHOST FOOD

In order for **LIVE-IT! 180°** to work for you, it's imperative that you move beyond what I call the "ghost food lifestyle." This lifestyle is built around the consumption of convenient, over processed foods – the kind you're probably used to buying in your local supermarket.

Moving beyond ghost food is achievable. That's a positive thing to consider. However, it will take time, effort, and energy for you to pull it off, because the structure of our society makes ghost food the default setting for most consumers. That's a big problem. *You and your accountability partner need to commit RIGHT NOW to eating less processed food – by which I mean food made out of refined and artificial ingredients – even though that food is convenient and comparatively inexpensive, or stop eating it altogether.* If you don't make that commitment, you are running the risk of major health problems.

"If you don't make this commitment, you are running the risk of major health problems."

The following major health problems are associated with eating processed foods:

Obesity. A 2012 study by the World Public Health and Nutrition Association links consumption of "ultra-processed" foods with obesity and points out that this category includes the five most commonly eaten foods in the United States: sweetened soft drinks, cakes and pastries, burgers, pizza, and chips. Obesity has been linked in clinical studies to any number of serious medical conditions, including stroke, high blood pressure, diabetes, cancer, gallbladder disease and gallstones, gout, Osteoarthritis, and asthma.

Heart disease. This is a clinically proven result of overconsumption of hydrogenated (trans) fats, which you can find in mass-produced ghost foods like doughnuts, cookies, crackers, muffins, pies, cakes, and French fries. I know – all the good stuff, right? No matter how good it tastes, no matter how tempted you are to ease these items into your shopping basket or place your familiar order in the drive-through, you and your accountability partner *must* make a commitment to eliminate hydrogenated fats from your daily consumption ritual. Why? Because these fats are some of the most heart-hostile substances you can put into your body. That's the truth.

Metabolism problems linked to refined carbohydrates. Not all carbohydrates are created equal. The kinds of carbs Big Food likes to use – the refined, pulverized, heavily processed kind – are very, very quickly broken down in your digestive tract. This means you get rapid spikes in your blood sugar and your insulin levels, followed by major carb cravings a few hours later when your blood sugar levels drop again. In addition to the metabolic problems caused by these foods, major consumption of refined carbohydrates has been shown to connect to any number of nasty chronic diseases.

A host of lethal health problems connected to the consumption of high-fructose corn syrup. In the decades since Big Food moved away from cane sugar and toward high-fructose corn syrup as its go-to sweetener, it's saved a lot of money. You know what else has happened? American food consumers have been experiencing elevated rates of hypertension, metabolic problems, type 2 diabetes, kidney disease, and non-alcoholic fatty liver disease. This is not to say that cane sugar is "good for you" in equally large quantities – it's not – but rather that Big Food, knowing that sweet foods tend to addict well and sell well, has opted for a cheap, addictive sweetener and is now using it on a massive scale ... a scale that is fueling a major public health crisis. Guess what? Big Food simply doesn't give a damn. They don't care about your health. So, you (and your accountability partner) must.

Ghost food may look like food, smell like food, be easy to buy, taste great, and seem like it has some

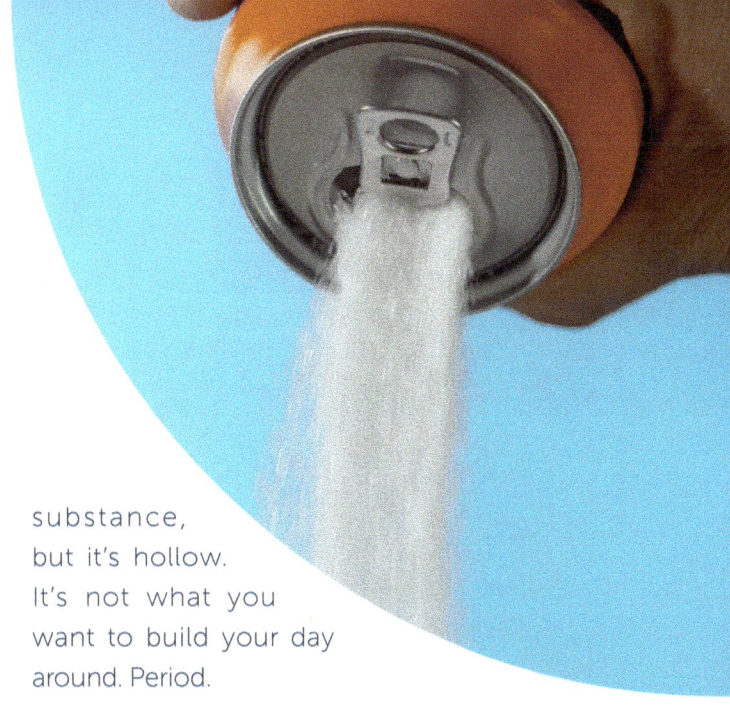

substance, but it's hollow. It's not what you want to build your day around. Period.

Here's the bottom line: Ghost food isn't just candy bars and soda – it's anything that's been processed in such a way that the nutrients have been degraded or removed and the addictive properties have been enhanced. And I'm sorry to have to be the one to break it to you, but that breaks down to *most* – not all but *most* – of what you are used to buying in your local supermarket. So that purchasing pattern needs to change.

At the end of this chapter, you'll find a Good/Better/Best breakdown of the ideal ways to make the changes to your food intake that you need to institute as part of **LIVE-IT! 180°**. Be sure to discuss these with your accountability partner, and be sure each of you choose, and support, a FUEL option you feel comfortable with.

Are these changes always going to be comfortable or familiar? No. Are they worth making anyway? Yes.

FUEL

LIVE-IT! 180° INSIGHT

It's way, way better to change a bad habit than it is to die early. And that applies to the habits that play out in your kitchen.

There is a lot of evidence that people fail to eat healthily simply because they're not prepared to do so, either psychologically or practically. Specifically, they have not done a full Kitchen Makeover.

In other words, they haven't gone through their kitchens and cleansed them of all the ghost food and junk that's in there. That's an essential part of this process for both you and your accountability partner. You will need to clean out your kitchen, because when we face adversity, we go back to what's familiar to us. That means in the middle of the night, if everything is still in the kitchen, the same way it was before we started **LIVE-IT! 180°**, we're going to reach for the ghost food. It's how we're wired. For now, just know that this change is a MANDATORY part of **LIVE-IT!** Don't worry right now about executing all the details of your kitchen makeover, just be aware that it's an integral part of the system and that you can't expect to complete the FUEL principle without doing it. (You'll learn more about the Kitchen Makeover in the Appendix.).

SOME ADDITIONAL THOUGHTS ON "WHAT WORKS"

The question that's probably on your mind right now is, "What the heck do I get to eat and when do I get to eat it?"

Let me ask you to put that question on hold for a moment. I want to share some of the critical things we've learned from implementing LIVE-IT! 180° successfully with people who had spent decades eating the way Big Food wanted them to eat – and who *did not* particularly feel like changing that pattern. (Remember that, not so very long ago, that was me too!) My goal here is to share with you *what works* ... and also to identify what doesn't.

First, here's what doesn't work: putting up a list of "good" foods and portion sizes on your refrigerator, memorizing that information, and then attempting to live up to it, without changing anything else about the way you eat. That leads to failure, so I beg you not to do it.

Here's what *does* work: changing not only the types of foods and the quantities of foods you eat, but also the *way* you eat. Let me briefly explain why this is so. Changing a pattern that's been ingrained for your entire life and that connects to something as fundamental as food is a big transition. You're probably used to eating in a certain way. Not only that, you're out to break an addiction. (Yes, much of the Ghost Food you can buy in the grocery story is literally addictive.) So, considering all that, you deserve the most powerful and effective best practices to support you as you make that transition. You deserve a behavioral plan that supports the change you're making.

Three best practices in particular will help you to make this change. These are three very simple behavioral changes you can do, starting right now, that will make it much, much more likely that you will succeed in implementing the eating changes I'm going to be sharing with you in this chapter. I call them BEHAVIOR SUPPORTS, and I'll break them down for you now.

BEHAVIOR SUPPORT #1: Eat slowly. Whenever you're eating, no matter what it happens to be, no matter how you're feeling, no matter whether you've had a good day or a bad day so far, I want you to *slow down*. That means chew consciously. Breathe consciously. Be mindful of what you are eating. *Notice* what you are eating. Don't find

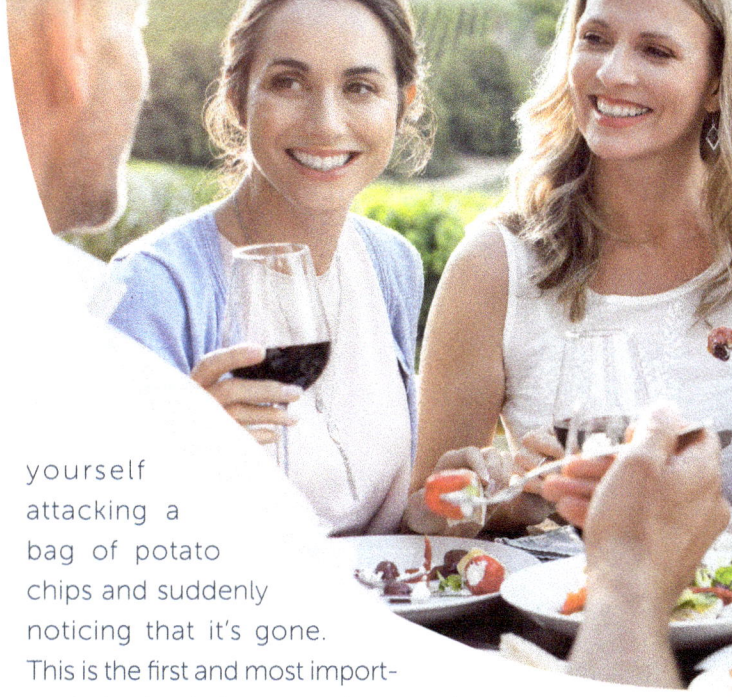

yourself attacking a bag of potato chips and suddenly noticing that it's gone. This is the first and most important behavioral change – take your time.

I want you to take 20 minutes to consume each main meal of the day, and I want you consume the food slowly. Why is that important? In 20 minutes, your body releases hormones that allow you to create a state called satiety (sa-TIE-uh-tee) – the feeling of being satisfied. Not full but satisfied. If you eat fast, it will take you 20 minutes to feel like you have reached this point. If you eat slowly, it will *also* take you 20 minutes to feel like you are satisfied. This is an extraordinary mechanism by Intelligent Design that has been set up within our bodies. Here's what it accomplishes: If you take your time and use the body's natural mechanisms to avoid pouring more energy into the system than the system can hold, less food will end up being stored in your body as fat.

85

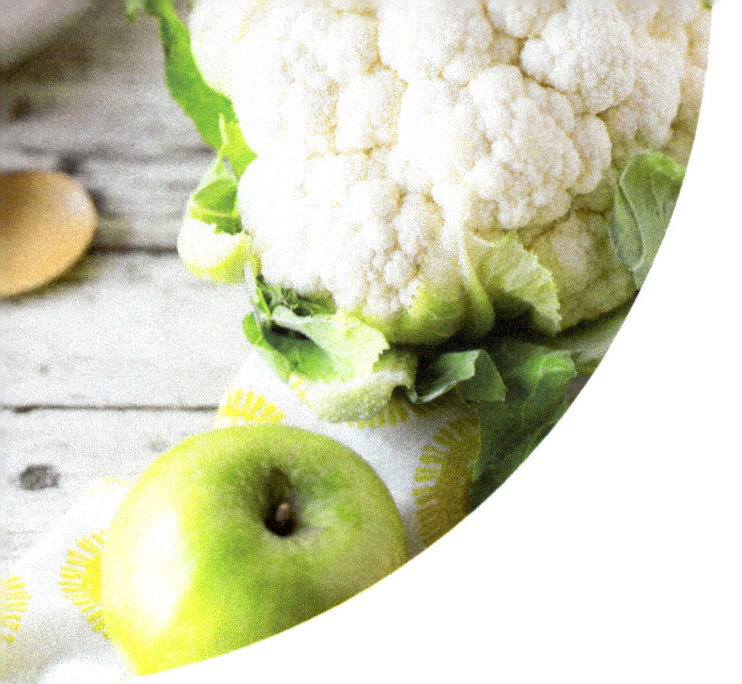

BEHAVIOR SUPPORT #2: Be in the moment. Simply put, this means *don't do anything else while you're eating* except socialize with the people who are eating with you. Notice them. Notice the food. Pay attention to what's happening. Don't distract yourself. For twenty minutes, set some in-the-moment ground rules as you and your family and/or friends eat together: no TV, no emails, no checking your phone, no video games. Take this time to notice the people you're with and to notice the flavors and textures of what you're eating. Do one thing at a time. Enjoy the food together (or enjoy food by yourself if you happen to be alone).

BEHAVIOR SUPPORT #3: Only eat to 80% of your stomach's capacity. You know that feeling of having taken in so much food that you "couldn't eat another bite?" I think we all do. That's known as being 100% full. Starting today, you're only going to get to four-fifths of the way there. You're going to stop overloading your body. You're going to leave a little bit of room in your stomach at the time you stop eating. This is not the same thing as leaving a little bit of room and then filling that space with some artificially sweetened Ghost Food dessert. I'm talking about *stopping the meal when you are satisfied, well before you feel full*. For some people, this takes a little practice. But after just one or two days of practice, you will know when to stop.

Please consider *all three of these behavioral supports to be mandatory*. If you and your accountability partner commit to them and execute on that commitment, you will succeed in making not just a *dietary* change (which typically does not last very long, regardless of our intentions), but a *lifestyle* change (which, if you do it right, can be both positive and permanent). Following the simple guidelines I've laid out for you will make it much easier for you to initiate *and sustain* that kind of lifestyle change. It will also reduce your stress levels by making it easier for you to move away from unhealthy eating patterns. I suggest you begin by adopting behavior support #1 for one week. Then add behavior support #2 in the second week and the last behavior support in the third. At the end of the three weeks, you may be very surprised at the outcome and benefits of these modified behaviors! If you continue following these three behavioral supports for a total of five weeks, you will be surprised to find that you have formed a new life-changing habit.

LIVE-IT! 180°: WHAT TO EAT, HOW MUCH TO EAT, WHEN TO EAT

In the system that you're about to learn, you'll notice that, instead of one or two big meals that strain your body's metabolism, I'm asking you to eat smaller meals and a maximum of two snacks each day (which you earn, spread out over the course of the day). There's a reason for this. People in today's society tend to fall into a cycle of starve and binge. For instance, they often skip breakfast, or skip breakfast and lunch, maybe "grabbing something" (like a doughnut or a candy bar) to "get them through the day." Then they eat their one main meal late at night.

This is bad for your body, because it misses the whole idea of eating quality food as the *fuel* that you need during the course of the day. Think about it. If you have a fireplace and you put a log on the fire at eight o'clock in the morning and then leave it alone all day long, what's going to happen? The wood will burn down and burn down, and when you get to eight o'clock at night, the fire will have gone out. If you want a steady fire that keeps burning all day (and I promise, you do), you will have to throw on a few more good logs during the course of the day.

The same principle applies to your eating habits. Your body's metabolism has to "keep the fire burning" throughout the course of the day. If you don't add a meal every three to five hours, your fire is going to start to die down. After a day or two of not feeding the fire (by adding fuel), your body starts going into a self-preservation mode by slowing down vital systems. If This is stressful. If you make a habit of straining your metabolism with starve-and-binge practices, your body is more likely to begin storing energy as fat so that it can deal with this self-preservation cycle. By Intelligent Design, if you don't convince your body that there is plenty of food available, it will starts to slow your metabolism down (which means you don't burn fat) and store any fuel you do send its way as fat. And that means you're going to gain some weight!

> *"Keep the fire burning by eating three meals a day – no exceptions."*

Starve-and-binge is a dangerous cycle to make your body follow. So, here's a better idea. Keep the fire burning by eating three **LIVE-IT! 180°** meals a day – no exceptions. Don't starve. Don't binge. Eat something every three to five hours. I've added the option of snacks to give you a little flexibility. If, after trying this for two weeks, you find that you are feeling hungry throughout day, this means you are burning energy, which is good. If you exercise strenuously for 30 minutes each day, in accordance with the DRIVE principle we'll be discussing later, you earn the right to the two snacks per day I mentioned above. (The details about specific quantities are below.) Ideally you should eat one of these snacks in between your morning meal and lunch, and the other in between your lunch meal

FUEL

87

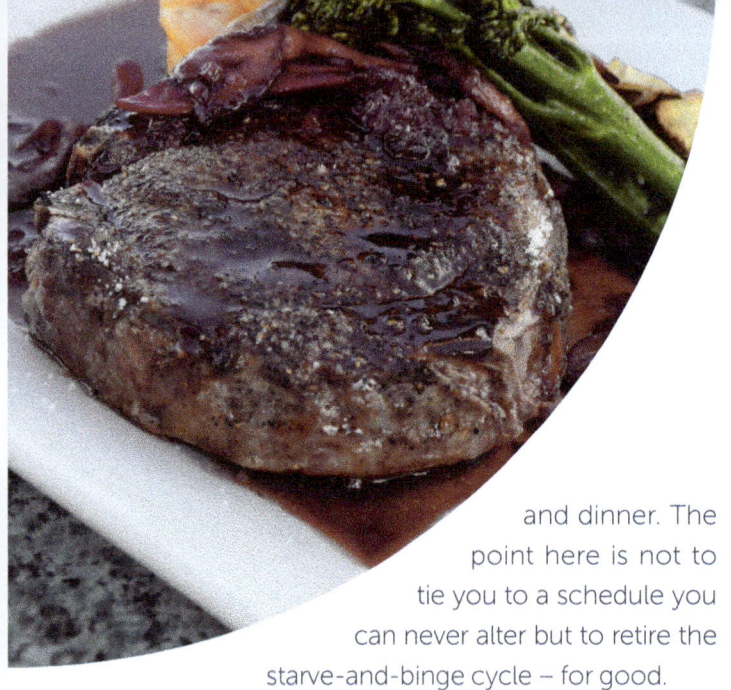

and dinner. The point here is not to tie you to a schedule you can never alter but to retire the starve-and-binge cycle – for good.

So that's what you need to know about timing. Next, let's talk about the quantities you'll be eating.

How do you determine how much you eat with **LIVE-IT! 180°**? It's really simple. You don't need scales, weights, or measuring cups, which may have confounded you in other "diet" plans in the past. With **LIVE-IT! 180°** – which, remember, is not a "diet" but a way of living – all you need is your body. You're going to be using *your own hand* as the primary measuring tool.

Here's why. At age five, whether you realized it or not, your hand was the perfect tool for you to use in determining how much food you should take in. At age 55, your hand is, of course, going to be bigger, but it's still going to be the right measure to determine how much food you should take in. That's how perfectly your system has been designed. Ok, so how does this work in reality, and how much should you eat at each meal?

PROTEIN

The first macronutrient we need to eat at every meal is **protein**. Whether it's animal protein or vegetable protein, the amount of protein your body has to consume in one meal is the *exact same size and width as the palm of your hand*. That doesn't include your fingertips. It's from the very top of your wrist to where the fingers begin.

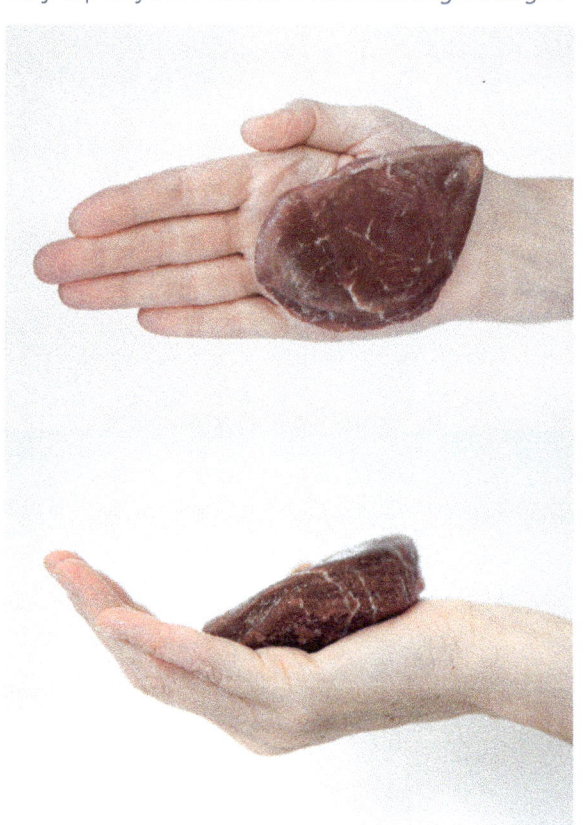

So, at every one of your three meals a day – breakfast, lunch, and dinner – you're going to give yourself one palm full of protein. By the way, protein is things like eggs, chicken, fish, beef, and pork –

LIVE-IT! 180° TIP

Big Food adds nitrates and nitrites to foods like bacon, salami, sausages, and cured sandwich meats to give their products an appealing color and prolong their shelf life. The problem is, both nitrates and nitrites can form nitrosamines in your body, which can increase your risk of cancer. Why is it legal for Big Food to do this? Because they have close relationships with the people who write and enforce the food laws! So, check the ingredients. If you see nitrates or nitrites, skip that item.

yes, even bacon or sausage, but this must be high quality pork with no nitrates/nitrites. If you don't eat meat, you can eat beans. However, read my caution about beans later in this chapter. I recommend getting your meats and all your pork from a local butcher if possible. If the pork that's available to you is the heavily processed kind that relies on nitrates and nitrites, you'll want to skip pork. (Note: Nuts are a protein, but I include them under fats. I also don't recommend peanut butter, for the simple reason that the peanuts used in peanut butter sometimes have quality and inspection problems, and because research has linked some cancers with peanut butter.)

There is an exception to this one-palmful-a-meal guideline when it comes to protein. If you are younger and you're very active, or you're exercising strenuously five or six days a week and you're burning a high calorie intake by elevating your heart rate for at least thirty minutes during each of those sessions, you are allowed *two* palms of protein per meal. Why? Because you're expending lots of energy. Again, you'll be learning more about this issue in the DRIVE principle.

Sometimes people ask me: "What if I'm not working out at all, but I want to enjoy those two palms of protein at every meal?" Here's my answer: Start working out! I'm serious. The act of elevating your heart rate five or six times a week will totally transform your relationship with food. Not only will you get the extra protein, but your feelings of hunger and your cravings for specific foods will recede ... eventually becoming a thing of the past. Try it and see.

VEGETABLES

Next, let's look at your **vegetable** intake. These are things like broccoli, carrots, cauliflower, zucchini, spinach, green beans, summer squash – every vegetable group, really, but not fruits like apples, oranges, and bananas. When it comes to vegetables, you want to mix up your colors, because the more you mix your colors, the better the balance of nutrients and antioxidants. For example, you might eat yellow peppers with green Romaine

FUEL

lettuce, white cauliflower, and red cabbage. Make a mixture out of that, and your body will benefit. You'll get the full array of vitamins and minerals you need. How much of this should you eat? *At least one whole handful of vegetables per meal – and that means filling up your whole hand – including the thumb, palm, and fingers – with raw vegetables.* If it shrinks down after you cook it, that's fine.

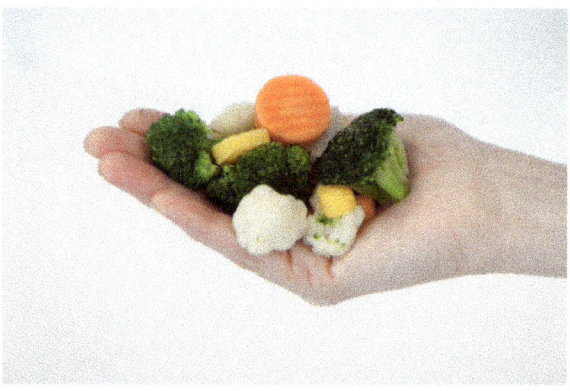

Notice that here, the one handful per meal is a minimum. You can eat two or more handfuls of vegetables per meal if you want, because most vegetables won't cause you to increase your weight and can only help you. So, feel free to chow down on those chopped carrots! One note of caution here: while *most* vegetables qualify for this two-or-more-handfuls-per-meal standard, starchy root vegetables, such as yams, potatoes, or squashes, don't. So keep those to one handful per meal.

GOOD FATS

Now let's talk about your intake of the so-called **"good fats."** I'm not going to bore you here with a long scientific discussion about what distinguishes a good fat from a bad fat, because a) it's pretty boring and b) I suspect you've already heard a lot of this discussion and tuned it out. Suffice to say that certain fats, when eaten in moderation and used to replace saturated or trans fats, can help you reduce your cholesterol levels and your risk of heart disease. You'll find those good fats in things like olive oil, almonds, nuts, and seeds. Coconut oil is a great good fat that I recommend be consumed every single day. It is a superfood in my book with a ton of health benefits. I could write a whole book on the benefits of coconuts. Check out the liveit180.com website for more information. I want you to eat one serving of these good fats at each of your three meals. How much should you eat at each sitting? Enough to equal the volume of your thumb, from the tip of your thumb down to where it meets your palm. Again, if you're engaged in an exercise program that equates to 30 minutes or more of strenuous exercise each day, you can double that to two thumbs' worth of good fats per meal.

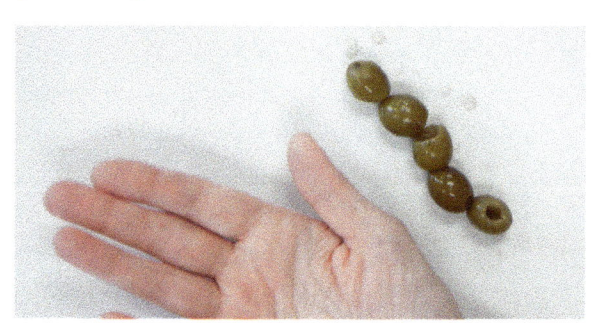

FRUIT

The last piece of the puzzle is **fruit**. In **LIVE-IT! 180°**, you are entitled to have no more than one cupped handful of fruit at *two* of your three daily meals. In fruit, there is more energy than there is in some other foods, and if you're not burning it, it's going to build up as fat. Here again, if you work out a lot, you can have three cupped handful-sized servings a day. Some people on **LIVE-IT! 180°**, who are working out regularly, save the third handful of fruit for a late-evening snack, teaming it up with the extra serving of good fats they earned.

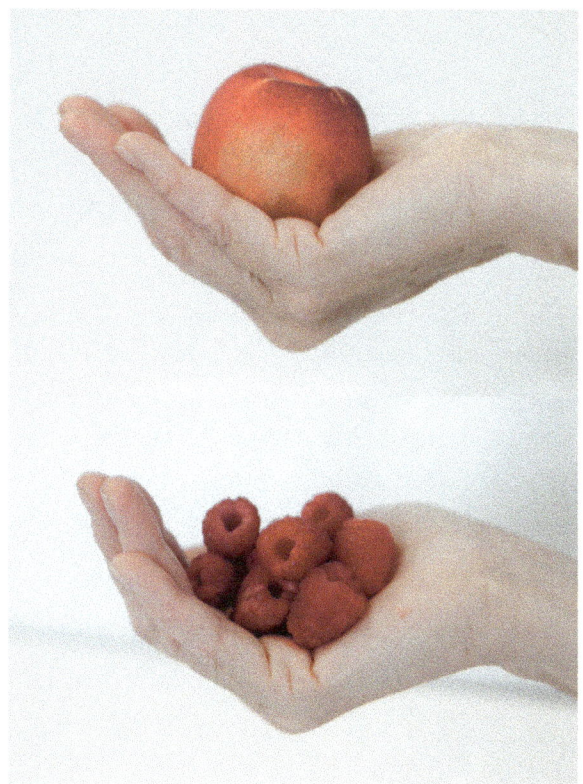

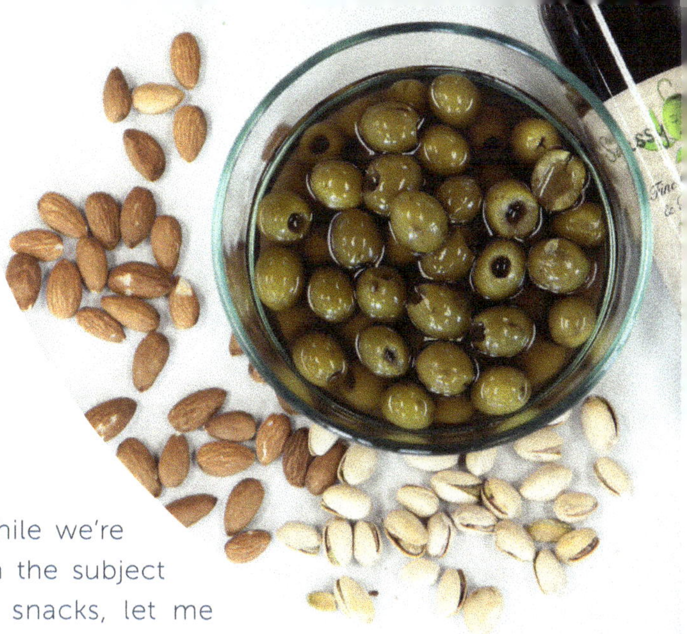

While we're on the subject of snacks, let me share with you another advantage of getting those daily 30-minute workouts in regularly. You can earn two snack meals a day. The first is an additional palmful of protein and a thumb of good fat, and the second is an additional palmful of protein and a handful of vegetables. These can be eaten anytime between meals, but I have found that there is a benefit to consuming these two earned snack meals around your workouts. Try to enjoy that additional palmful of protein and a thumb of good fat before your workout, and the additional palmful of protein and a handful of vegetables afterwards. (I recommend sweet potato, which is a great food for rebuilding strength after a workout.) Of course, you don't have to eat these two snack meals unless you feel like it. Remember that you will need to plan out your other three meals for the day for every three to five hours, to make sure you keep the fire burning.

1st SNACK

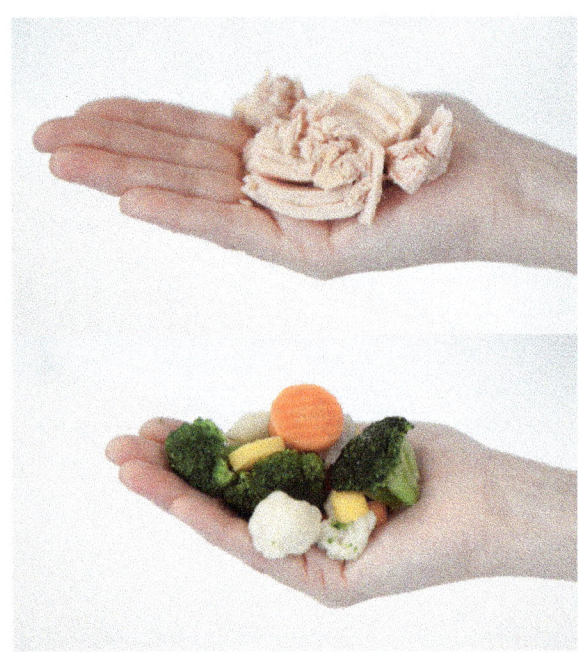

2nd SNACK

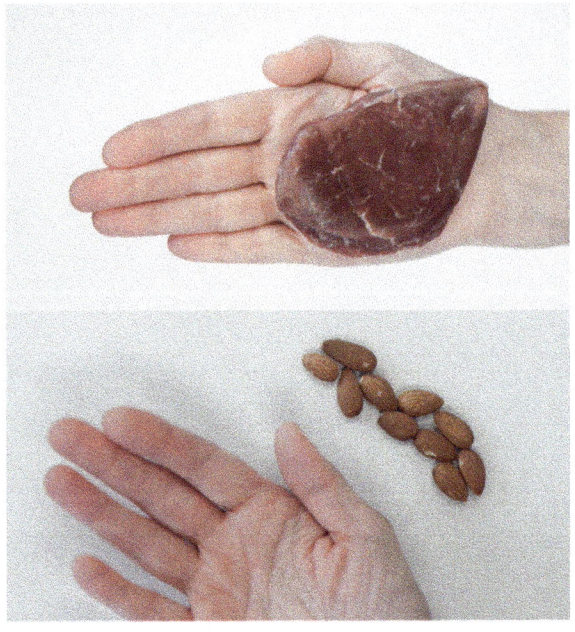

WATER

Of course, you need to drink plenty of **water**. As I mentioned a little earlier in this book, the amount of water you need to drink is "half your body's weight" in pounds – by translating the pounds into *ounces* of water. In the example I gave earlier, a person who weighed 200 pounds would have to drink 100 ounces of water each day. This simple change will have a dramatic positive effect on your metabolism, your energy level, and your outlook on life. *Most of what makes up your body is water. Make sure you up your water intake to the level recommended here, according to your total body weight.*

I realize that just focusing on the food categories and the quantities can seem a bit restrictive. But once you learn the system and get familiar with it, you'll discover for yourself that *it's really not about following rules*. It's about training your body to attain higher energy levels and perform at peak levels. And it's about enjoying yourself in the process. Translation: You're going to have fun with this! I've included some ideas in the Appendix that I think will help to make this transition an enjoyable one for you and your accountability partner.

A FEW WORDS ABOUT DAIRY

When looking at the "hand system" of portion measurement I just described, many people ask "Where's the dairy?" The answer is – it's not there.

I'm not saying you must instantly eliminate all dairy products from your life. I am saying you need to transition out of a dietary pattern that is based on over-reliance on dairy products. I realize this may be difficult for you, because lots of us have been trained for a very long time by Big Food (of which Big Dairy is a powerful component) to consider milk, cheese, yogurt, and all the rest of those products to be an essential part of a healthy diet. They are *not* an essential part of a healthy diet unless you happen to be a recently born calf.

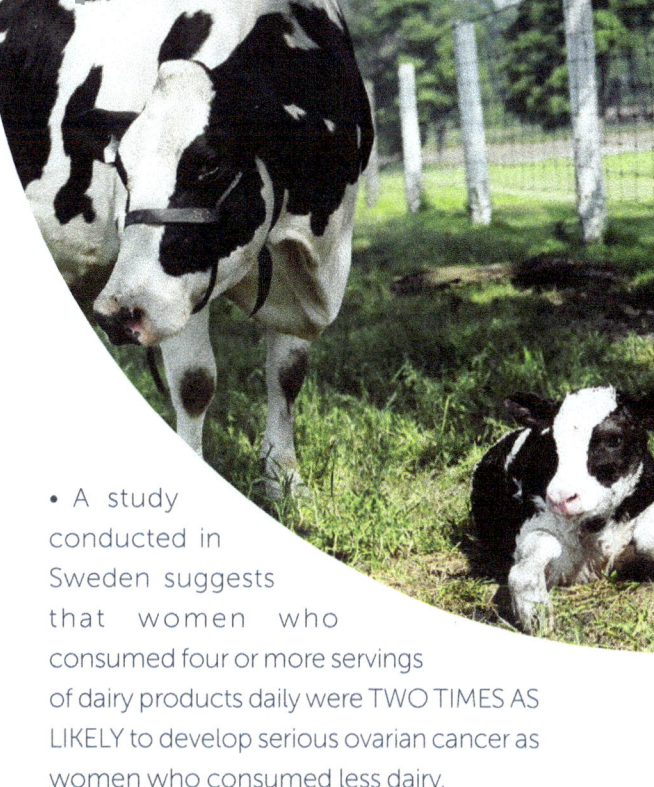

Consider the following:

- Even though the powerful pro-milk lobby has been telling us for decades that milk builds strong bones and strong bodies, a recent medical study showed that women who drank large quantities of cow's milk every day were MORE likely to sustain fractures than women who drank little to no milk.

- Some studies link ingestion of dairy products with increased risk of prostate cancer for men. On a similar note, there is evidence that a low- or no-dairy diet reduces the incidence of this kind of cancer.

- Cow's milk has a sugar called lactose that is so difficult for some people to digest that they experience gas, nausea, cramps, and diarrhea. Lactose intolerance is not a disease. It's your Intelligently Designed body telling you something.

- A study conducted in Sweden suggests that women who consumed four or more servings of dairy products daily were TWO TIMES AS LIKELY to develop serious ovarian cancer as women who consumed less dairy.

- Many cows, including most of those Big Dairy uses to give you milk, are heavily dosed with hormones and antibiotics. Bad news. Believe me when I say you don't want that stuff in your system.

I could go on with the scientific data, but you get the idea. Suffice to say that I speak from personal experience when I tell you that even small amounts of milk may cause long-term negative health effects. The phlegm and congestion you get when you drink milk is not normal. It's your body telling you, *Hey – I'm not a calf!*

Let me also point out here that the milk you can buy in most grocery stores has been processed and "fortified" to such a point that it is nutritionally meaningless. Add it all up, and what you have is

FUEL

A FEW WORDS ABOUT GRAIN

It comes as a big surprise to some people to learn that there is virtually no grain consumption built into the ideal ("Best") **LIVE-IT! 180°** eating routine.

This whole program first came into being because I was concerned about the systematic inflammation and related serious health issues that I was experiencing personally, problems that I knew, as a health and nutrition coach, had to have something to do with the food I was eating. I did a lot of research into this question, and what I learned alarmed me. It was this: **The modern American diet is built around massive overconsumption of something that the best authorities know for certain isn't good for us and that I know for certain is not meant to be part of our Intelligent Design when it comes to food consumption: grains.**

Put bluntly: We were not designed to eat anywhere near as much grain as society suggests we should. Most of us don't know that. Why not? Well, there are a lot of reasons, but in large measure I believe it's because there are significant economic downsides (from Big Food's point of view) to having a populace that is well informed about the serious health problems that scientific studies have linked to excessive consumption of grains.

This means that we should "swim against the current" by educating ourselves and taking appropriate action when it comes to grain consumption.

LIVE-IT! 180° INSIGHT

t's not a question of how MUCH grain consumption is likely to damage your body.

The truth is, we don't know how LITTLE will damage your gastrointestinal system over time.

That's why you need to get on the trajectory of eliminating grain from your kitchen.

a scam by Big Food to sell you something that is not needed by your body and has the potential to hurt you.

At the end of this chapter, I'll share some insights on how to make the transition from dairy dependency. In the meantime, rest assured that you really *shouldn't* think of this as another thing you "have to give up." There are plenty of great milk alternatives that will help you with the transition.

> "Big Food sells you something that has the potential to hurt you!"

Please understand: I'm not saying grains are inherently evil, and I'm not saying you have to immediately eliminate them from your plate or bowl, starting today. What I'm saying is that we need to recognize that Big Food controls, in large measure, what the food supply looks like in this country, and that government (in the form of the Food and Drug Administration) tends to confirm that control. As a result, most of us have been raised to believe that consumption of grains is the "base of the pyramid" or one of the major "food groups" we need to be sure we consume every day. **This is false, and we need to challenge it.** I say that with some emphasis, because the best current research indicates that:

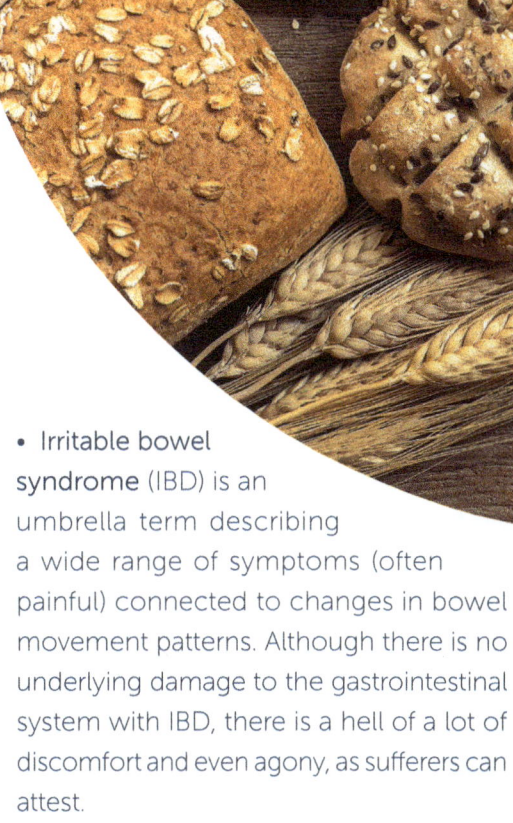

- Grains contain anti-nutrients (including, but not limited to, gluten) that can and do hurt the human body. Some people's bodies repair this damage better than others, but there's really no sane reason to do the damage in the first place.

- Specifically, these anti-nutrients have been shown to cause and/or worsen the conditions known as Crohn's disease, irritable bowel syndrome, and leaky gut syndrome.

- **Crohn's disease** is a serious, debilitating, inflammatory bowel disease that can affect any portion of the gastrointestinal tract, from the mouth to the anus.

- **Irritable bowel syndrome** (IBD) is an umbrella term describing a wide range of symptoms (often painful) connected to changes in bowel movement patterns. Although there is no underlying damage to the gastrointestinal system with IBD, there is a hell of a lot of discomfort and even agony, as sufferers can attest.

- **Leaky gut syndrome** is exactly what it sounds like: tiny holes in your gastrointestinal system that let substances such as undigested food, bacteria and metabolic wastes leak into your bloodstream. It's very bad news, and there's a growing body of evidence suggesting that it's caused by eating foods (namely grains and legumes) that literally punch holes in your "straw."

So. If you don't want to punch holes in your straw (intestine), and I suspect you don't, then I'm going to ask you to take a good, close look at the guidelines for grain consumption that follow in the

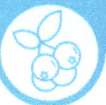

Good, Better, Best section of this chapter – and then follow those guidelines.

Let me repeat. **Grains, eaten in excessive quantities, punch holes in your gut, and whether or not you have experienced this for yourself up to this point, there is no good reason to hasten the day when you do.**

I should say that one of the big reasons I'm taking the time, effort, and attention to emphasize this point as intensely as I've done here is that I have personally experienced in my own life, and seen first-hand in the lives of many other people, including people I love, the deeply destructive impact that needless consumption of grains can have on human health. For me, this is personal. If you routinely eat a lot of grain, I want you to know that habit is dangerous. It's like taking a Brillo pad to your large intestine. If you don't believe me, Google the phrase "grains and chronic inflammation" and see what comes up. Also fascinating is "grains and autoimmune disease."

I believe there will come a day when the medical and governmental establishment is much more open and direct when it comes to challenging Big Food on this issue and will take appropriate action, just as it did in challenging Big Tobacco about the dangers of smoking. Until that day comes, the reality is that we are all on our own, and we all need to start making better choices about grain consumption. **LIVE-IT! 180°** is here to help you do that.

I want to assure you that there is plenty of time for you to adjust to this ideal routine. Moreover, you are not "wrong" or "bad" if it takes you a little time to adjust.

> "Grains, eaten in excessive quantities, punch holes in your gut."

A FEW WORDS ABOUT SUGAR

Be honest. Did you read that headline and think "My God, is he ever going to stop?"

Well. Yes. I am. This is my last Ghost Food target for this chapter. Does that help?

I realize I'm running the risk of sounding a little bit like a critical parent here, taking aim at all your favorite foods. I also realize that maybe, right about now, you're thinking to yourself that there's no more fun to be had with a spoon and fork. But I can promise you that's not true. Please consider these two points. Point one: You're going to have a lot more fun and a lot more energy once you have adopted the **LIVE-IT! 180°** approach to eating (and sleeping and moving and socializing and decompressing) for a couple of months. And point two: If you care for someone, you tell them the truth. I really do care about what happens to you and your accountability partner. So ... here's the truth Big Food would rather you didn't know about sugar:

- Most Americans eat three or four times more sugar than the government's current best guess of how much is healthy. Much of that sugar consumption comes in the form of cheap high-fructose corn syrup, which is used in countless processed food products, and which I've talked about earlier in this chapter.

- Specifically, the average American consumes 82 grams – six teaspoons – of sugar each and every day. Eating that much sugar (whether you spoon it out and stir it into your coffee, or eat it in the form of heavily processed food that contains too much high fructose corn syrup) leaves you open to the following health problems:

  » **Liver damage** - in some cases, comparable to that which an alcoholic would experience.
  » **Heart disease** - with significantly shortened life expectancy.
  » **Kidney disease** - with significantly shortened life expectancy.
  » **High blood pressure** - also known as hypertension. This, too, can dramatically impact your life expectancy.
  » As if all of that weren't enough… Sugar turns into fat and feeds the bad bacteria in your system. That means your body has to work harder than it should to fight off infection … at the same time you're gaining weight. Not good.

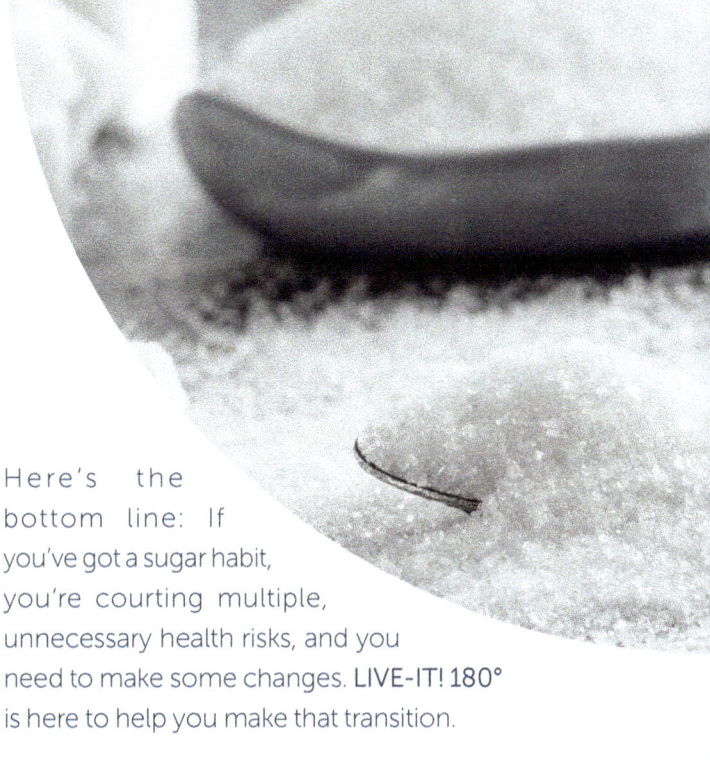

Here's the bottom line: If you've got a sugar habit, you're courting multiple, unnecessary health risks, and you need to make some changes. LIVE-IT! 180° is here to help you make that transition.

THE SUPPLEMENTS CONTROVERSY

It will probably come as no surprise to you to learn that the medical establishment has taken a very dim view of food supplements in recent years and of the entire industry that produces and markets those supplements. People often ask me if I've heard about all the negative feedback that food supplement producers get from medical organizations and from countless media outlets. The answer I give always seems to come as something of a surprise to them. I say: "Yes, I have read that negative feedback … and on the whole, I agree with it."

This usually generates a surprised look.

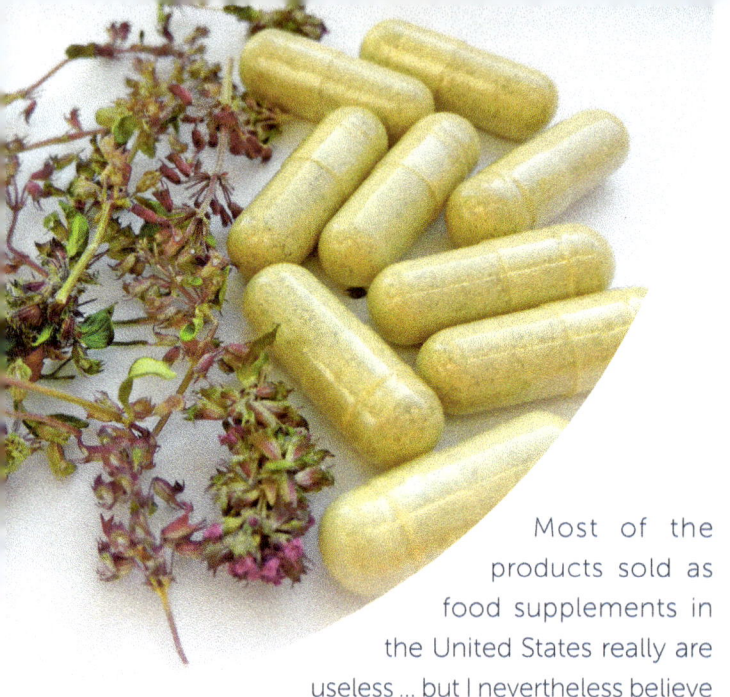

Most of the products sold as food supplements in the United States really are useless ... but I nevertheless believe you should add supplements to your daily FUEL plan. The reason for that is pretty simple. It's true that the vast majority of supplement products out there are junk. But *not* all of them are junk!

Here's my experience. By picking the right supplements, I put myself on the right track, much more quickly than I would have otherwise. You can do the same, if you avoid the junk and pick the right supplements. First, you need the lowdown on why you are, in all likelihood, best advised to throw away any and all supplements you bought at the local supermarket or pharmacy.

Because of the way most food is manufactured today, the raw materials that supplement producers use to create their products are laden with chemicals and pesticides. This harsh fact – combined with the synthetic, bottom-line-driven, nutrient-hostile processes that these companies use to meet production quotas – degrades and ultimately neutralizes the nutritional value of whatever it is they're pumping into the pill or capsule and then selling to you.

The result: You're paying good money, and sometimes quite a lot of it, for something that simply doesn't work and doesn't add any value to your day. Period.

"The vast majority of supplements are junk, but not all of them are junk."

So yes, the doctors and the investigative reporters are right. Most supplements on the market today are worthless. They're a complete waste of your time, money, and attention. But I can tell you from personal experience, and a whole lot of research, that more reputable providers create supplements that deliver significant nutritional advantage. *Their process, which is woefully under-represented in the marketplace right now, is based on something called whole-food constitute.*

Whole-food constitute supplements are not the synthetically re-created "product" that shows up in the bottles you typically find in the local supermarket. Whole-food constitute supplements are authentic, unadulterated, organic nutrients that are delivered to you without any kind of over-processing or chemical manipulation. They show up in the pill just the way they show up in natural foods. This means that your body is far better able to absorb and use these nutrients.

> ### "NUCLEAR STRENGTH": What does that mean?
>
> "Similar to the principles on which Viagra raises your main sail, (L-arginine) increases the body's production of nitric acid, which is proven to help maintain erections, according to the journal Neurology. 'It relaxes and widens blood vessels,' says Jayney Goddard, President of the Complimentary Medicine Association, 'which means your penis gets a better, more consistent supply of blood.' Giving you a better, more consistent supply of sex ... Nuclear strength – don't expect much shut-eye with this one:"
> – Men's Health
>
> January 1, 2018, issue.
>
> http://www.menshealth.co.uk/sex/your-penis/natural-viagra-226765

Think of "traditional" vitamins as being man-made and chemically-driven, in the laboratory, from ingredients that are sadly tainted by modern production methods. Think of whole-food constitute supplements as being responsibly processed organic nutrients that come straight from the farm to you, without pesticides and without shortcuts.

They're the real thing. They use organic ingredients that have been generated at the plant level, and not in a laboratory somewhere. That makes what you're taking in actual food – complete with all the enzymes you need to absorb and process the nutrients – rather than a chemical substitute. My experience is that whole-food constitute works.

FOUR DAILY SUPPLEMENTS

Let's get started. At a minimum, you will want to incorporate supplements from the following four categories.

A daily supplement that takes your gender into account - Men need different kinds of nutritional support than women do. That means they need different daily supplements.

If you're a woman who has not yet experienced menopause, you will want a supplement that helps you to replenish the iron that's lost during menstruation. In addition, you'll want the standard range of vitamins, in whole-food constitute form, including Vitamin B (to support cardiovascular function, healthy energy production and nervous system health) and vitamin D (to support healthy bones and mood functioning). You'll also want things like cranberry and chaste tree berry (which support a healthy response to changes associated with normal hormone fluctuations). Note that drinking sweetened, commercially produced cranberry juice is a net loss from the point of view of giving your body what it needs. If you are a woman going through menopause, or who has already experienced menopause, there are potentially a lot of issues at play, including maintaining support for healthy bones. Visit us at www.liveit180.com and check in with us so we can help you identify the right daily supplement for you.

If you're a man, you'll want a supplement that's been formulated without iron, because iron is not recommended for men unless it has been specifically recommended by a healthcare practitioner. Here again, you'll want a daily supplement of whole-food constitute vitamins. In particular, you need B vitamins (to support cardiovascular function, healthy energy production, and nervous system health) and vitamin D (to support healthy bones and mood). You also need zinc (an essential mineral, to support good prostate health).

Please notice that each of these supplements should include healthy doses of Vitamin D, which is essential and all too often overlooked, especially during the winter. We get Vitamin D from the sun, but a shortage of Vitamin D when you're indoors a lot, or when it is cloudy for long periods of time, can lead to Seasonal Affective Disorder, a serious llness.

Note: What I'm advocating here are just the basic requirements for men and women. Depending on your situation, you may require additional nutrients. Check in with us at www.liveit180.com and we'll help you find the right mix.

Probiotics - Whether you are male or female, you'll also want to take a good daily probiotic. This is important because our large and small intestines contain lots and lots of bad bacteria. We have to have bacteria in our intestinal tract to break down food, but the bad bacteria that builds up in our system over time can cause a whole bunch of bad conditions that can lead to diseases in the intestines, systematic inflammation, and autoimmune dysfunction. A probiotic will help you to build up the good bacteria in your system, so these good bacteria can get to work destroying the bad bacteria, helping with the absorption of nutrients, and promoting healing in your intestinal tract. But there's a catch: The good bacteria must be *alive* in order to do their job! Many of the probiotics out there fail this simple test, because of the bottom-line-first way they're manufactured. As a result, they're useless.

A daily Omega-3 supplement - This is best taken as a liquid, in the form of fish oil, because you don't want anything added to the mix, and you want to ensure that what you take is fresh. Omega-3 fatty acids have been clinically shown to help prevent and manage heart disease and may help to lower blood pressure.

Daily consumption of turmeric - Turmeric, a staple spice of Indian cuisine, has been around for centuries. It contains curcumin, a substance that carries potent anti-inflammatory and antioxidant properties. I strongly recommend that you buy it in bulk, keep it on your table right next to the salt and pepper, and season your food with it. (I bet you'll like it!)

HOW TO GET HOLD OF THE RIGHT SUPPLEMENTS

So. Those are the basics. You can buy the turmeric anyplace that sells good Indian-food ingredients. I strongly recommend that you buy the Omega-3 fish oil fresh (we can help you find that), and that you get the daily supplements from MegaFood, which is the only supplement producer I trust. Check in with us at www.liveit180.com and we'll get you started with the right products.

Whatever you do, please remember this: *Spending money on the overprocessed, nutritionally dead food supplements you are likely to find on the shelves of your local supermarket or pharmacy is a mistake. Don't do it!*

AND NOW, A WORD ABOUT L-ARGININE

L-arginine is a chemical building block called an "amino acid." The body uses it to make proteins. It's found in red meat, poultry, fish, and dairy products. It has been used successfully to treat a wide range of heart and blood vessel conditions, including congestive heart failure (CHF), high blood pressure, and coronary artery disease. It's also used for senile dementia, blocked arteries, erectile dysfunction, and male infertility.

I'm not saying every man should be taking L-arginine on a daily basis, and I'm certainly not prescribing it to treat any medical problem ... but I am suggesting that men at least consider looking into the list of benefits, which is long and impressive. For my part, I can only share my own experience with L-arginine, which has been entirely positive. I had an irregular heart rhythm – I was born with it. For years, this was something my doctor was concerned about. I started taking L-arginine on my own initiative, having done a little research on it. A few months later, during my regular checkup, my doctor was absolutely flabbergasted to find that the heart problem had simply corrected itself! I don't know the precise details of the cause-and-effect relationship, but I know I'm glad I started taking L-arginine daily, and I certainly wouldn't want to stop now. Not after my doctor looked me in the eye and said, "You've got the heart rate of a sixteen-year-old!" (I was in my mid-thirties at the time.)

L-arginine's status as the primary "natural Viagra alternative" – recently confirmed by *Men's Health* magazine – is also worth taking into account if you or someone you love is concerned about erectile dysfunction and/or male menopause symptoms.

AND NOW, A WORD OR TWO ABOUT THE HUNGER GAME

Let's face it, we live in an instant-gratification world. Let's say we're at home with our partner, and we decide we want to relax on the couch and watch a movie. What happens? We hit a couple of buttons, and the movie comes up on our smartphone or computer. Or suppose we want to talk to a friend as the movie's playing. What do we do? We pick up the phone, hit speed dial, and in a second or two we're talking to that person about the film. The response isn't just limited to entertainment and communication, though. When we're watching that film and our body sends us a signal that says "Hey, I'm hungry," what do we do? We take a similar instant-gratification approach. We pause the film, head over to the fridge or pantry and get ourselves a bag of potato chips and a container of cookies (or whatever it is we're used to). Then we head back to the sofa with our partner and hit "play." All too often, we look down, and the chips and cookies are just … gone.

There are times when an instant-gratification response works against us. One of those times is when we instantly answer our body's "Hey, I'm hungry" message with a plate of food (even good food). We need to change that pattern, because the body often tells us it's hungry when it's actually got all the fuel it needs. We need to train it to send us that signal a little less often. And you know what? With the help of an accountability partner, we can.

You may feel skeptical about that or even feel as though I'm asking you to do something that's impossible. I promise, it's not impossible. If you're eating three meals a day, and the two snacks we've talked about, and your partner is not only supporting you in that effort but actively joining in, you will quickly find that your body *isn't* hungry from the standpoint of actually needing nutrients and energy. The reality is, before you make **LIVE-IT! 180°** a way of life, sometimes you hear that "I'm hungry" message because other things make you long for food – like stress, lack of social connection, or even boredom. Those experiences are making your body send you a message that *sounds* like hunger but isn't. In short, the instant-gratification stimulus-and-response pattern, which has built up over decades, is playing a game with you, a hunger game. To make **LIVE-IT! 180°** work, you need to take enough time to recognize that game for what it is.

Let me make you a promise about hunger – if you stick with the hand-size meal approach I've laid out here for six straight weeks, and if you get support from your accountability partner, you will find that hunger quickly recedes as a problem for you. You are retraining your body. You are giving it a new pattern to follow. Give it a chance to adjust. The hunger pangs will eventually come under control. In the meantime, *you won't die* by waiting for your next meal or snack. I can promise you that, too.

People who follow **LIVE-IT! 180°** faithfully, with a coach or accountability partner, or via LiveIt180.

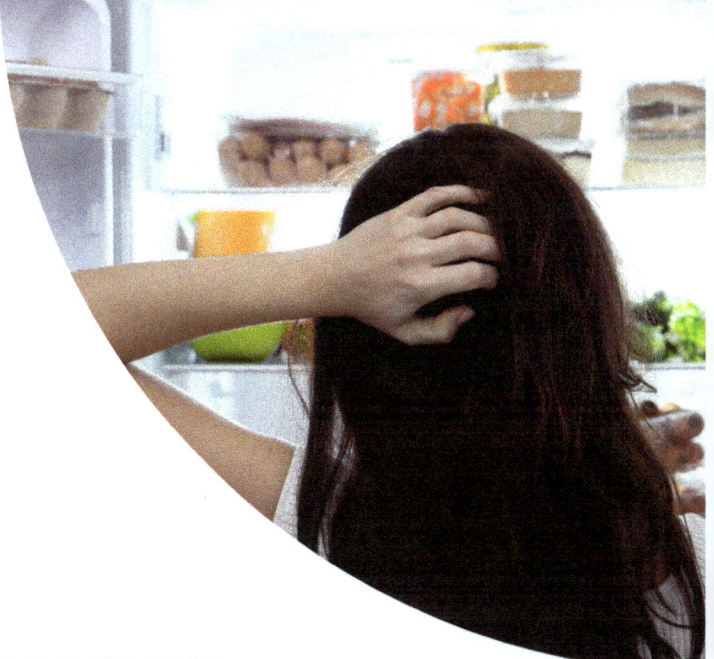

com, typically reach a point after just a few weeks where they say, "I'm not really hungry. Is it really time to eat already? Oh, okay. Let's eat." Give yourself time to get to that point. When in doubt, have a cup of tea. Or work out! It's easier than you think to ride out the hunger pangs. They really will disappear if you remain committed, stick to your plan, and stick to what works. I know you'll be glad you did.

GOOD, BETTER, **BEST**: PERSONALIZE LIVE-IT! 180°

Finally, it's time to see what this all looks like in action.

Not everyone will approach the FUEL principle of **LIVE-IT! 180°** in the same way or with the same degree of discipline. Just as you did in the RECHARGE chapter, you're going to discover there are multiple ways to do this "right." So please notice that this is a dynamic model, meaning that there is likely to be movement between the phases over time. You may start out at GOOD, move your way up to BETTER, get all the way to BEST, and then slip back down to BETTER. That's okay. Just make sure you stay on the system. If you happen to fall off the wagon, climb back on.

Here's how it breaks down.

"GOOD" – PHASE ONE

At this stage, you're simply following the basic system I laid out for you earlier in the chapter. Follow the guidelines I shared with you in the WHAT TO EAT, HOW TO EAT, WHEN TO EAT section, being careful to follow the advice on water consumption. Check out a concise, easy to access summary of what I shared with you previously at the end of this chapter.

People have lots of questions at this stage, including:

- **Do I have to throw away any foods that aren't mentioned in WHAT TO EAT, HOW TO EAT, WHEN TO EAT?** No. Give yourself two weeks to consume all the stuff that's in your pantry right now. Yes, you read right: You don't have to throw away any of the Ghost Food that's already in your possession. Go ahead and finish it off ... just know, as you do so, that you're saying goodbye. This is the initial, and probably the most important, phase of your Kitchen Makeover, which is discussed in Chapter Ten, and covered in much greater depth in the Appendix. Use this two-week transition period to get used to following the "hand portion" measurement system. Supplement that system with whatever Ghost Food you feel like eating. The one qualification here is: During this two-week transition period (which, by the way, is the only one you'll get as part of Live-It!180°), I want you to start *noticing* how much sugar, high-fructose corn syrup, and grain you are consuming. Discuss these levels with your accountability partner. You might also want to keep track of this information by recording it in a journal.

- **Does that mean I can I eat as much sugar as I want to at the GOOD stage?** No. It means you get to be the judge of how much sugar and high-fructose consumption you feel is appropriate. I'm not here to tell you exactly how much that is, *but* ... the amount you consume should be less than it was in the first two weeks.

- **Do I get to consume as much dairy as I want?** The approach to dairy is very similar. I want you to notice the level of dairy you consumed during the first two weeks and reduce that to a level you feel you can live with. You get to be the judge of how much your own dairy consumption goes down... but you do need to make sure it goes down.

- **What else changes after the two-week transition period?** Here at the GOOD stage, you can continue to consume rice, bread, pasta, and other grain-based products, as long as you cut your consumption of these products IN HALF, compared to what you ate during the first two weeks. After that, you will look for more ways to reduce your grain intake over time. For instance: If you were eating grain products at every meal, aim to make at least one meal a day grain-free.

- **Anything else?** Yes. Be sure to share all this information with your accountability partner.

"BETTER" – PHASE TWO

Congratulations! You're doing great. Now it's time to build on everything you accomplished in the "GOOD" phase and take your game to another level.

Much of what you've grown used to will stay exactly the same. As in the GOOD stage, you are going to observe all the "hand-based" portion guidelines I shared with you in the WHAT TO EAT, HOW TO EAT, WHEN TO EAT section. And as in the GOOD stage, you're going to make sure you follow the advice on water consumption, which is crucial.

In addition, you're going to start to change your buying habits. Specifically, you're going to start buying fruits and vegetables labeled "organic" – which basically means grown without synthetic pesticides, chemical fertilizers, or genetic modification. At the very least, you're going to be purchasing organically grown:

- Apples
- Strawberries
- Grapes
- Celery
- Peaches
- Spinach
- Sweet bell peppers
- Nectarines
- Cucumbers
- Cherry tomatoes
- Snap peas
- Potatoes

These "dirty dozen" items are your priority when it comes to organic purchases because, at the time of writing, their mainstream, non-organic equivalents are the most likely to have major problems with pesticide residue. (By the way, you may be able to find a more up-to-date list. Just Google the phrase "dirty dozen vegetables" and see what comes up.) It may be possible to get organic options for these fruits and vegetables at your local supermarket. More and more big supermarket chains are bowing to the increased demand for pesticide-free produce, which is definitely a good thing.

A side note: Please be sure to buy all your fruits and vegetables *in* season, no matter where you shop. Produce that shows up radically out of the expected season (apples in early February in New England, for instance) has typically been flown in from some other country with a potentially less reliable definition of "organic" or other problematic quality issues.

If you want, you can continue to buy non-organic equivalents of fruits and vegetables that don't make the "dirty dozen" list.

At the BETTER stage, I also want you to begin checking the ingredients of the food products you buy. So, if you look at the label and you find more than seven ingredients, or even *one* ingredient that you find hard to pronounce, please put that product back on the shelf and pick out a replacement with seven or fewer *pronounceable* ingredients. In addition, you're going to avoid all processed foods. Yes: That means you aim to eat only fresh foods. Nothing in a can. Nothing frozen. Nothing with preservatives.

Questions people typically have at this point about the BETTER phase include:

- **What about sugar and high fructose corn syrup?** Reduce your consumption of these to between 45 and 60 grams per day. Assume that your fruit consumption contributes 15 grams of that.

- **What about dairy?** Eliminate dairy from your world. You can replace it with a daily glass of almond milk or coconut milk if you want.

- **What about grains?** At the BETTER stage, you're going to limit your grain consumption to fresh corn and brown rice. Supplement the WHAT TO EAT, HOW TO EAT, WHEN TO EAT guidelines with *one palm* of either of these grains at *one* meal a day. This must include NO bread or other product made from wheat or wheat flour. If you want, you can replace this additional grain serving with bread or pastry made from coconut flour, almond flour, or cashew flour.

- **Is that it?** Nope. One more change. You should reduce your caffeine intake to a level that represents HALF of the caffeine you were consuming in the GOOD stage.

As with the GOOD stage, share your experiences and insights about the BETTTER stage with your accountability partner.

"BEST" – PHASE THREE

Ready to move to the top tier of the FUEL plan? Great! Here's what that looks like.

Continue to follow the "hand-based" portion guidelines I shared with you earlier, being sure to follow the guidelines on water consumption. In addition, shift to buying *only* organic produce and meat. Again, this means you are choosing *not* to put synthetic pesticides, chemical fertilizers, hormones, antibiotics, and GMOs into your system. Good call! (If you want an eye-opener about what Big Food pumps into the assembly-line meat most people eat, visit http://bit.ly/hormones_antibiotics) Make it your goal to stay as close to the ground as you possibly can with your food choices.

Here at the BEST stage, you're going to get even better at checking the ingredients. If you look at the label and see more than *five* ingredients listed, or even one ingredient that you find hard to pronounce, you need to put that product back on the shelf and pick out a replacement. Five or less to thrive! As with the BETTER stage, you're going to skip all processed foods. To clarify, that means nothing in a can, nothing frozen, and nothing with preservatives.

As with the BETTER stage, you must avoid all dairy products. You can opt instead for a daily glass of almond milk or coconut milk.

The most common questions I hear about the BEST stage are:

- **How much sugar and high fructose corn syrup can I eat?** Here the top tier, you must reduce your consumption of sugar and high fructose corn syrup to below 45 grams per day. Assume that your fruit consumption contributes 15 grams to that total.

- **How about grain?** Ideally, there is zero grain consumption at this level. Yes, you can do it. I promise. And your gastrointestinal system will thank you for it. Feel free to use recipes with coconut flour, almond flour, or cashew flour for occasional snacking. If you absolutely insist on a once-every-two-weeks exception to this, treat yourself to a muffin and a couple of pieces of toast.

- **And caffeine?** At the BEST level, drink no more than one cup a day. Go decaf if possible.

A quick overview of a daily meal plan at the BEST stage is at the end of this chapter.

Here's my guarantee: If you and your accountability partner change your patterns and adopt one of these three options, making **LIVE-IT! 180°** your daily routine for six consecutive months, you'll both have so much more energy, joy, and possibility in your life that you'll never want to go back. And you won't miss anything you've "given up."

When in doubt, remember that this is not about pretending there are magical "good foods" and demonic "bad foods." It's about avoiding the most obvious eating hazards, setting the right trajectory, and adopting a responsible, informed lifestyle you can sustain over time.

"You are what you eat." —Michael Pollan

Plan your life and live your plan. LIVE-IT! 180°.

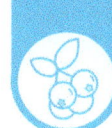

THE LIVE-IT! 180° DAILY MEAL PLAN

Breakfast

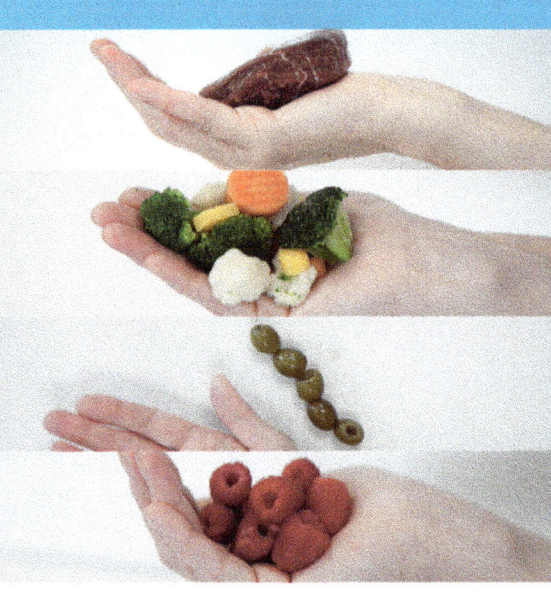

- ✓ 1 palm of protein
- ✓ 1 whole hand of veggies
- ✓ 1 thumb of good fat
- ✓ 1 cupped hand of fruit

Mid Morning Snack
(if earned from working out)

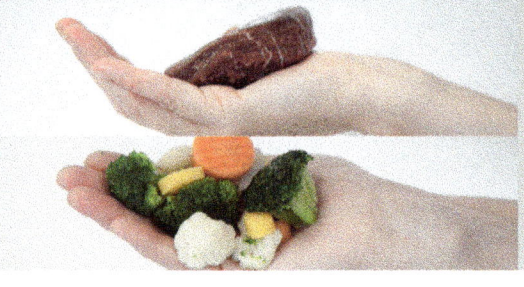

- ✓ 1 palm of protein
- ✓ 1 whole hand of good veggie carb (i.e., sweet potato)

Lunch

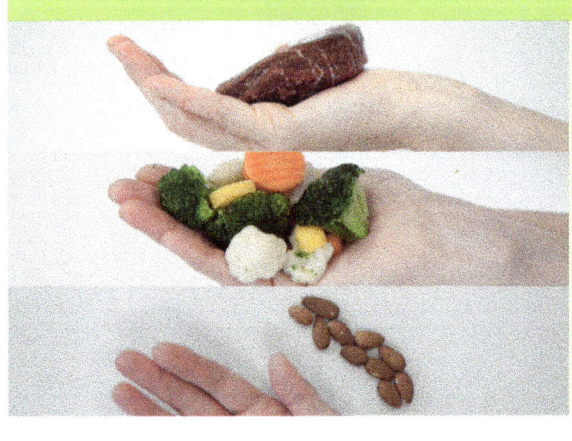

- ✓ 1 palm of protein
- ✓ 1 whole hand of veggies
- ✓ 1 thumb of good fat

Afternoon Snack
(if earned from working out)

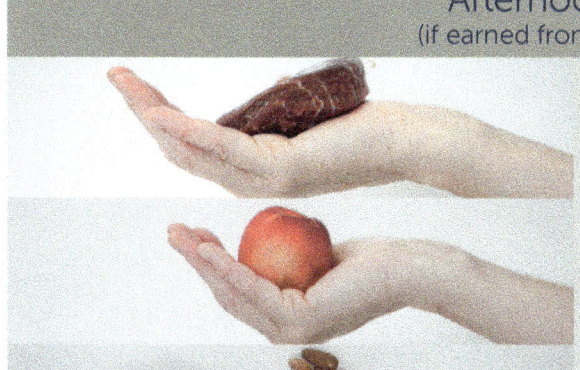

- ✓ 1 palm of protein (optional)
- ✓ 1 cupped hand of fruit
- ✓ 1 thumb of good fat

Dinner

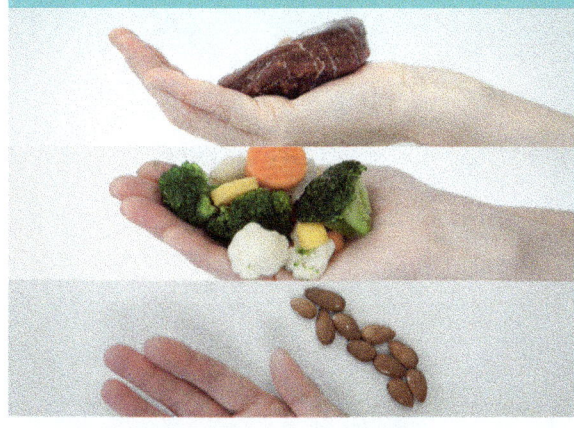

- ✓ 1 palm of protein
- ✓ 1 whole hand of veggies
- ✓ 1 thumb of good fat

Evening Snack
(if you didn't have the afternoon snack)

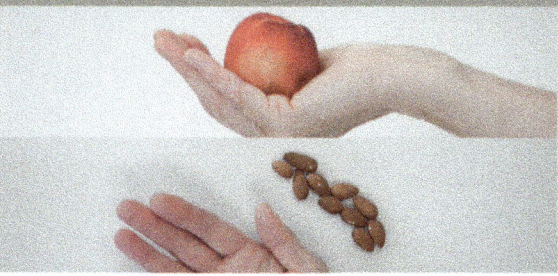

- ✓ 1 cupped hand of fruit
- ✓ 1 thumb of good fat

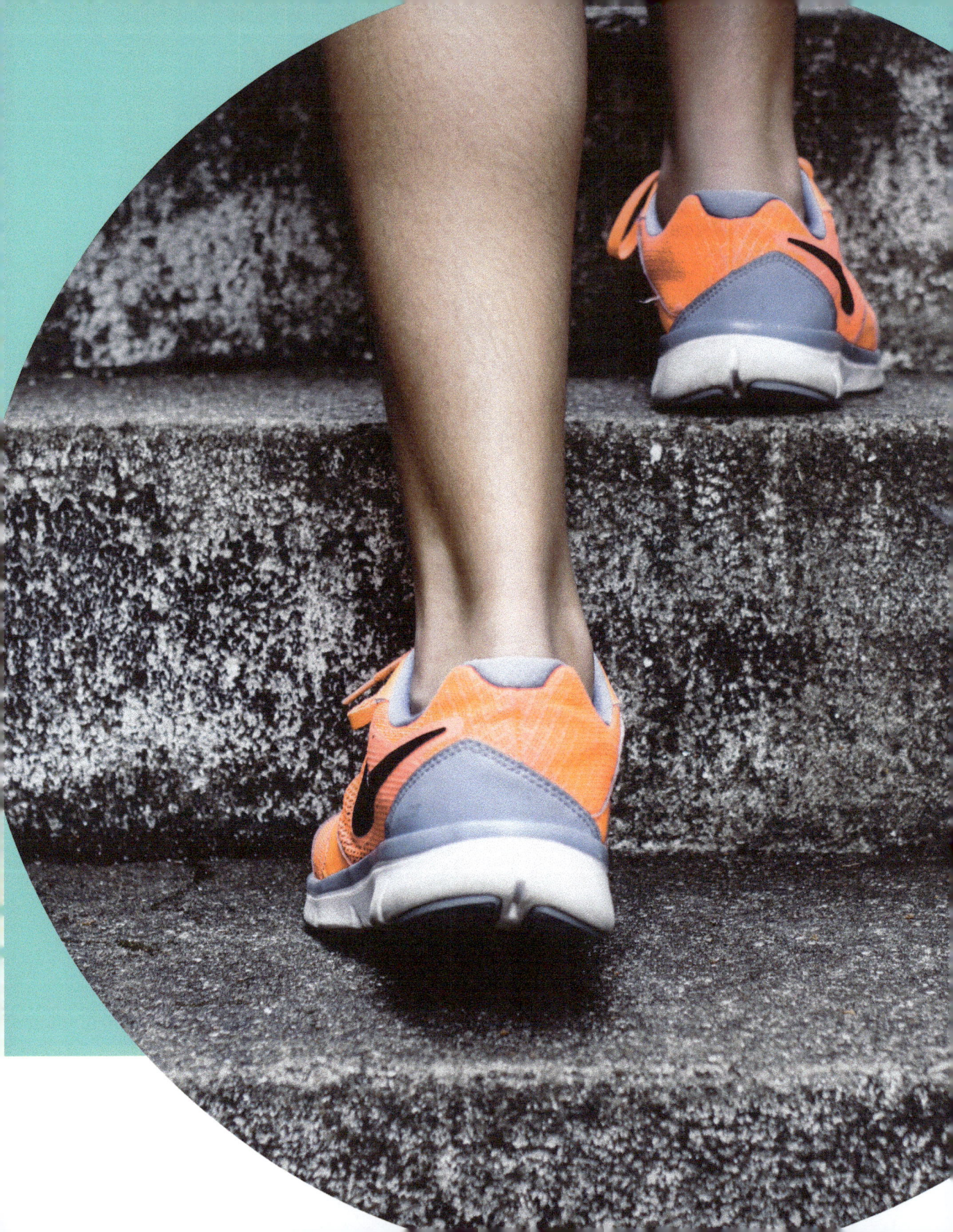

DRIVE

Move your body regularly by actively using it. Exercise is not a four-letter word.

7

You have to move your body regularly (by actively using your body)

Earlier, I asked you to think of sleep as the battery that starts your car and of food as the fuel that powers that superior, Intelligently Designed car. In this chapter, I want to ask you what your supercar is *meant* to do? The answer is simple. It's supposed to be brought out on the road. The battery is charged. The gas is in the tank. You're not going to leave it sitting unused in the backyard or driveway for weeks or months on end. If you did, the car would not be in very good running order when you eventually had to go somewhere. For a high-performance automobile to function properly, *you have to start the engine and drive it around on a regular basis*. If you don't do that, the systems are going to degrade and performance will decline, until eventually the car doesn't work at all. The same is true of the Intelligently Designed machine that is your body. In the immortal words of the Rolling Stones, *you've got to move*.

"You've got to move!"

THIS CAN BE AN EMOTIONAL ISSUE!

A lot of people become agitated when I talk about DRIVE. They bring a lot of baggage to the topic of EXERCISE, which is a dirty word as far as I'm concerned.

I'm not an impossible personal trainer barking out instructions and making people feel like they can't possibly keep up. I'm not a drill instructor shouting DROP AND GIVE ME TWENTY – or whatever else you were once pressured into doing by peer pressure or some authority figure. I'm simply talking about incorporating more movement into your day and building on that, day by day. You'll recall the baseline I set up for you earlier in this book: **Get out and walk for between 15 and 30 minutes each day.** To begin with, I want you to make sure you keep doing that. if you feel like expanding it a bit on your own, that's great, and that's up to you.

At the end of this chapter, you're going to find the same GOOD/BETTER/BEST behavior models that you saw in chapters Four and Five. These will help you to expand whatever you're doing right now in terms of DRIVE, but I want to beg you not to think of any of these best practices as the "E-Word." Doing that is likely to summon up all kinds of negative emotions, based on experiences

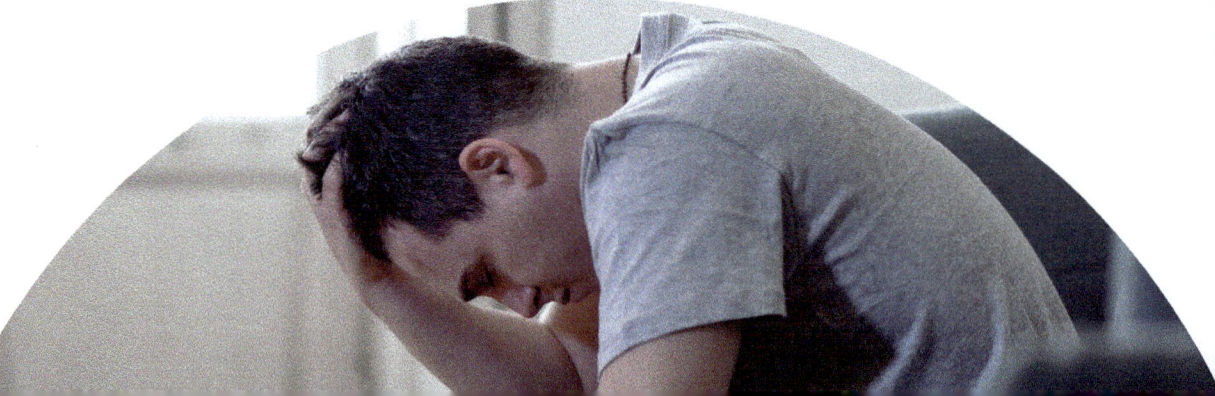

you've had in the past. This is all about a new *future* you're building for yourself and about the habits that will support that future. Get out of the pattern of thinking of the DRIVE chapter as something you are being made to do. These are your choices and your behaviors. YOU are taking control. Think of DRIVE as what you do every day with your supercharged, Intelligently Designed vehicle. You'll end up in a much better place.

WHY THIS IS SO IMPORTANT: THE SLUDGE FACTOR

Movement is critical to improving your overall lifestyle. It's an integral part of **LIVE-IT! 180°**.

That's me talking, of course, and what I say is less important than what you decide and what you do. *You're* going to be the one who changes your behavior pattern, and let's be honest, some of those changes may take a little more focus and a little more commitment than you've leveraged so far in your daily walks. Therefore, it's worth finding out why it's so essential to expand and build on what you're currently doing in DRIVE.

Your body is *designed* to move. Movement is what burns calories and fat. Moving strengthens our muscles and bones and our immune system, and specifically it strengthens your lymphatic system. It gets all your fluids moving so your joints, muscles, organs, bones, digestive tract, and finally your cells get the good stuff they need and eliminate

> ### LYMPHATIC SYSTEM: What does that mean?
>
> According to Merriam-Webster, the lymphatic system (also known as the lymph system) is "the part of the circulatory system that is especially concerned with scavenging fluids and proteins which have escaped from cells and tissues and returning them to the blood, with the removal of cellular debris and foreign material, and with the immune response." The system's job is to return essential fluids and proteins back to the blood and to destroy bad stuff (like bacteria) that is foreign and potentially harmful to the body.

the various by-products of life. Lubrication is so important for a healthy you! Without the right lubrication ... your body is subjected to what I call the "sludge factor."

Here's the interesting thing about your lymphatic system. **It only functions with movement.**

That's how your body was designed. If you have a very sedentary lifestyle with little movement, the watery fluid traveling between your cells and your tissues, known as lymph, is just as stagnant as you are. If sitting around watching TV for twelve hours a day becomes a sustained pattern of behavior, the lymph gradually turns into a kind of sludge.

The waste just sits there and coagulates. If you think of a stagnant pond with scum on top of it, that's a good illustration of what happens to your lymph if parking yourself in front of a TV or computer becomes a consistent lifestyle choice. It's just kind of nasty.

That's a problem, because the purpose of the lymphatic system is to remove waste from your cells and tissues and clean up your bloodstream. It's also there to take out dead cells and move nutrients around into your cells and tissues. Therefore, a stagnant lymphatic system is a major obstacle to your health and well-being.

LIVE-IT! 180° INSIGHT

Broadly speaking, the more you move, the better a job your lymphatic system is going to do, the more effective your immune system is going to be, and the stronger and happier you are going to be.

Movement, in short, is a major quality of life issue. As far as LIVE-IT! 180° goes, expanding the DRIVE profile is non-negotiable.

The reason movement doesn't happen easily or automatically for some people is that they get used to a pattern of inactivity. Then they experience physical discomfort as they try to move out of that zone of familiarity. (For instance, they may get headaches.) There are two big reasons this happens: First, people try to do too much, too quickly; and second, they don't approach their own lifestyle holistically. In other words, they focus on physical activity ... but ignore issues like whether they're getting enough sleep.

If you follow the guidelines laid out in this chapter, you'll avoid both problems. Also remember that the sludge, when it starts to get moving again, may cause you to get nausea, headaches, and dizziness. This is a normal part of the transition back to a healthy lifestyle. It means the junk is being filtered out of your system. (Always check with your doctor before beginning any movement program.)

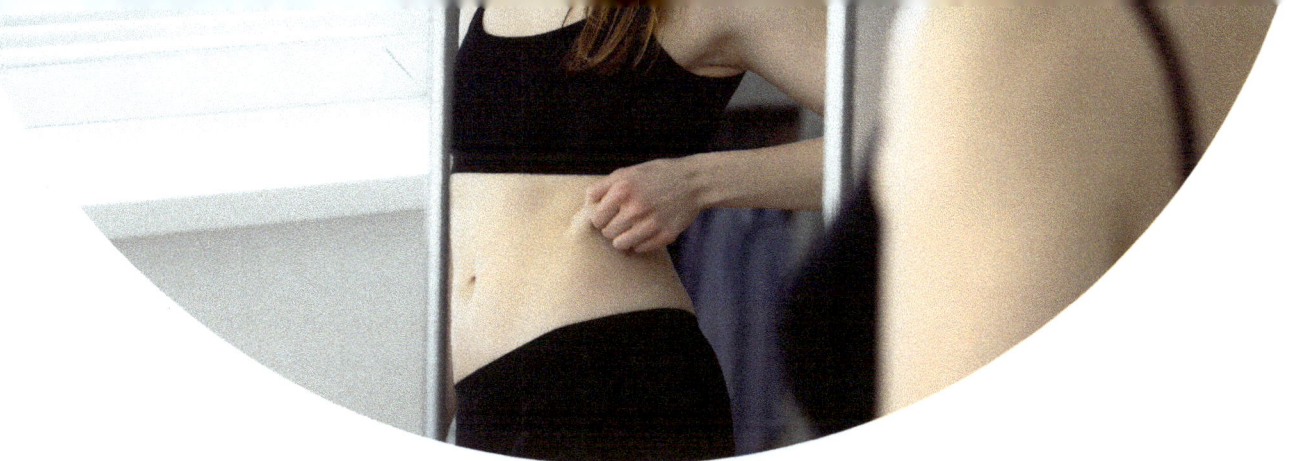

THE "MENTAL SLUDGE FACTOR"

There's something distinctive about the DRIVE principle that is different from the other elements we've been looking at. We are talking about moving the body, but the movement of your body inevitably depends on the movement of your mind. Your mental conditioning has a huge impact on the quality of the workout you get or whether you get a workout at all. If you don't control how you *think* about the DRIVE principle, you're likely to find yourself dealing with what I call "mental sludge," which is just as disgusting and just as dangerous as the physical sludge that builds up in your bloodstream. Here's the insidious thing: Most people don't even realize how mental sludge builds up. So, I want you to know what it is, how it happens, and what you can do about it.

Let's say you're getting out of the shower. You catch a glimpse of yourself in the mirror, and you notice that you've put on a few pounds over the past couple of months. Here's a question you may not have considered before. How do you respond to that realization internally?

If you're like a lot of us, you start a little conversation with yourself. It might sound like this:

Wow. I need to do something about that extra weight. I need to start a workout routine.

Yeah. I really do.

I wonder if my wife/husband finds me less attractive now...

You get the picture. On and on this discussion goes, and it *sounds* like it connects to something positive, starting or continuing your workout. This is the challenge: That kind of dialogue, if we choose to indulge it, is just a downward spiral. It ends up eroding our self-concept. It makes us think less of ourselves and our own potential. And – weirdly – it's addictive. We may even pick it up as a kind of mantra:

I need to work out.

I need to work out.

DRIVE

I really need to work out.

But the more we repeat that mantra, the *less* likely we are to get out and move! This negative mental cycle is a self-perpetuating barrier to physical activity of almost any kind. We add little variations to the mantra and begin an avalanche of self-pity that intensifies the longer we indulge it ... and keeps us from taking action.

I really need to work out. I'm fat.

I really need to work out. I'm old.

I really need to work out. I'm unattractive.

> "This kind of internal dialogue always makes it harder to take action."

As we repeat that mantra and find new ways to express it, we reinforce a sedentary lifestyle that has plenty of time for television and the Internet, but no time to get out and take a walk. This is mental sludge. It's the language of depression and incapacitation. It's the language of immobilization. It's the negative internal dialogue that blocks out positive energy and keeps us from working out.

The thing that makes mental sludge so dangerous is that whenever we engage in it, we tend to *think* we're doing something positive. Reminding ourselves of the need to work out. Offering a little helpful criticism that makes it easier for us to get out and do something.

Wrong. What we're really doing is lowering the chance that we get up off the couch! For some reason, indulging this kind of internal dialogue *always* makes it harder to take action and get moving.

More than any other element of **LIVE-IT! 180°**, the DRIVE principle is prone to this distinctive mental self-sabotage. We need to notice when we use our powers of internal communication to paralyze ourselves. We have to change our way of thinking about ourselves, our bodies, and our potential. We have to recognize mental sludge when it shows up ... and *instantly* take *constructive action to counteract it*. That constructive action can, in my experience, take one of three forms:

1: Do something physical, on your own, that you enjoy. This could be hopping on an exercise bike or heading out for a walk or dropping and doing twenty pushups. It could be anything really, as long as you get a kick out of it and do it right away, the moment you find yourself thinking, "I'm out of shape" or "I have to work out." One of the coolest things about DRIVE is that it makes negative internal cycles much more difficult to sustain.

2: Educate yourself. You could read a fitness magazine or watch a fitness video ... or even come back to this book and reread something that's meaningful to you.

3. Reach out to your accountability partner and share what's going on in your world. This doesn't have to be a lengthy check-in, and it doesn't have to sound like a therapy session. All you have to do is check in on how the person is doing on his or her DRIVE goals ... and share how you're doing with yours.

Mental sludge is crippling, but the good news is you can build up a response that beats it and takes it out of your system. Whenever you notice mental sludge accumulating, pick one of those three activities I just shared with you… and you'll do a much better job of protecting yourself from the *physical* sludge that can build up in your bloodstream.

THE MOST COMMON FORMS OF PUSHBACK

As I pointed out earlier, I get some very emotional reactions from people when I suggest that they take a more active role in expanding their daily DRIVE habits. Most of these, to be frank, are excuses designed to defend the relatively sedentary lifestyle that's most familiar to them. Here are some of the most popular forms of pushback I receive ... and the "reality check" answers I've used to begin a deeper and more productive discussion about the DRIVE principle. We all have these excuses, especially when we start to change our behavior patterns in a certain area. The first step is to recognize them for what they are, excuses. Then we can begin to

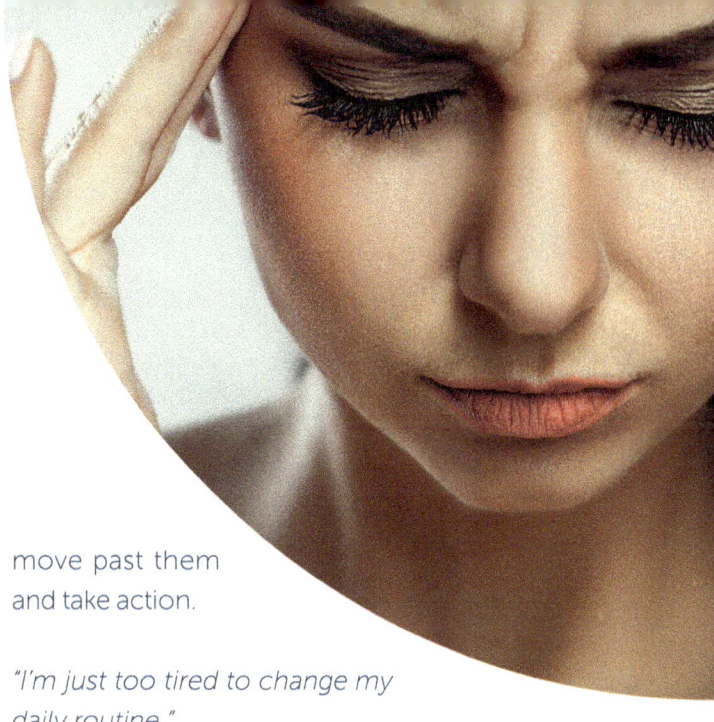

move past them and take action.

"I'm just too tired to change my daily routine."

A lot of people tell me this as they begin **LIVE-IT! 180°**. They've withdrawn all the available energy from the bank; there's nothing more left in the account. They'd like to do more movement, but they're too exhausted with everything else that's going on during the course of the day.

Reality check: It sounds persuasive, from a distance ... but it doesn't match up with the way the human body works. The very best way to get *more* energy is to *expand* your DRIVE behavior plan over time. If you stick with it and transition from a sedentary way of life to a more physically active one, you will soon find that you have more energy than you know what to do with ... and you will get a lot more accomplished.

"I've tried working out and didn't get any positive results."

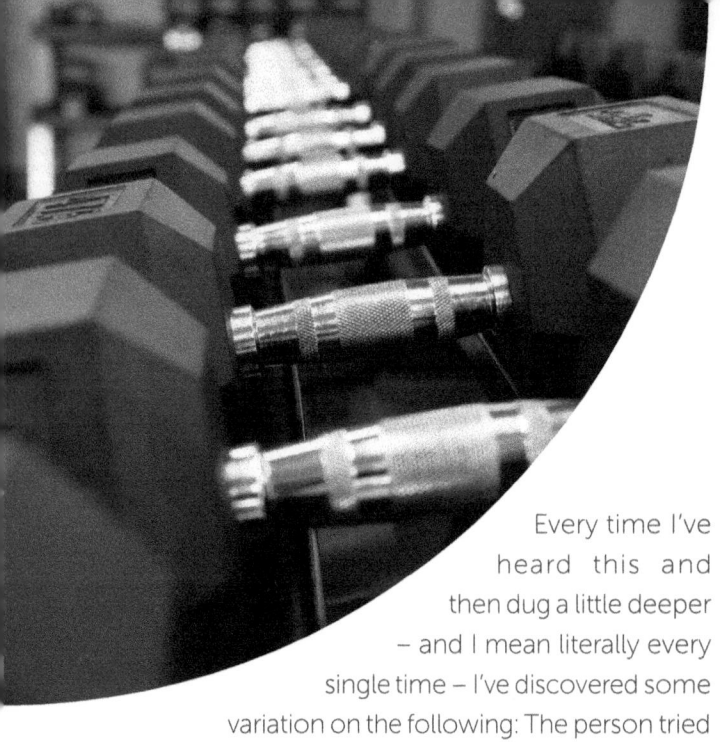

Every time I've heard this and then dug a little deeper – and I mean literally every single time – I've discovered some variation on the following: The person tried working out for a week or two, didn't see an instant transformation, and gave up.

Reality check: Here's my advice: *Stop thinking in the short term.* Stop checking in to see how you're doing. All the experts say it takes on average 6 to 8 weeks of sticking with a good workout routine to begin seeing even minor results. If you stick with something for that long, believe me, something good is going to happen to you. Don't worry about when it's going to show up or what it's going to look like. Just pick what you like to do from the GOOD/BETTER/BEST menu you'll find at the end of this chapter, do it in a daily basis, and leave it at that. Act and let the results take care of themselves. Don't worry about whether you're losing weight, don't worry about whether you're getting stronger, don't worry about anything. Just give it an honest chance. If you stay the course, you will get results.

"I've had bad experiences with working out in the past."

People who offer this response remind me of people who resist re-entering the dating scene because of one bad relationship experience. Instead of asking, "What made that experience the wrong one for me?" they ask, "How can I ever avoid having to experience any pain again under any circumstances?"

Reality check: Pain is part of life; the only truly serious challenge comes when you don't use the discomfort to learn and grow. In the case of DRIVE, it's important to understand that if you've been sluggish or inactive for a long period of time, you're going to have some physical symptoms as you re-engage your lymphatic system and start to get the sludge and the toxins out of your body. That's likely what you were going through with the "bad experience" you had in the past. Don't let that bad experience keep you from experiencing the joy and resourcefulness that is your birthright! Get the pain of the transition period out of the way – and move on with your life.

I can't emphasize it enough: Just doing one of the elements of **LIVE-IT! 180°** is not enough. That's why this hasn't worked for you in the past. If you don't have all the elements of the house built properly, your house will collapse! You need all five pieces of the puzzle in place for any one of them to function at the maximum level. Most people who push back on the *DRIVE principle have not yet attempted a holistic approach to physical activity.*

"I'm way too busy."

This is basically saying, "I'd love to – but my schedule is just too full. I've got so many commitments and so many things on my to-do list, I simply don't have the capacity to accommodate any more activities during the day. Not one more thing. I wish I could!" These people *are* usually also too busy to do things like show up at their kid's recitals. Their argument sounds reasonable, from a distance, if you don't think about it much.

Reality check: Think about the high-achieving people you've met – I mean the ones who truly inspired you and made you think, "That's who I want to be like." Were they physically active? I'm guessing the answer is yes. Did they get more done during the day than you typically do? Again, I'm assuming your answer is going to be yes. Do you think there's a possible cause and effect relationship there? The answer is yes.

All the studies have shown, and my own personal experience confirms this, that people who work out at least once a day are far more productive than people who don't. They get a lot more done. So, the real-world response here is: Your feeling of being too busy – and the added feelings of stress and of being overwhelmed – are a symptom, not a cause. They're a sign that large chunks of your life aren't working the way they should. To change that pattern, you need to reclaim your right to the energy, the clear thinking, and the breakthrough levels of personal productivity enjoyed by people who use safe, smart workouts to raise their heart rates and apply good stress on their muscles on a daily basis. That will fix the problem of being

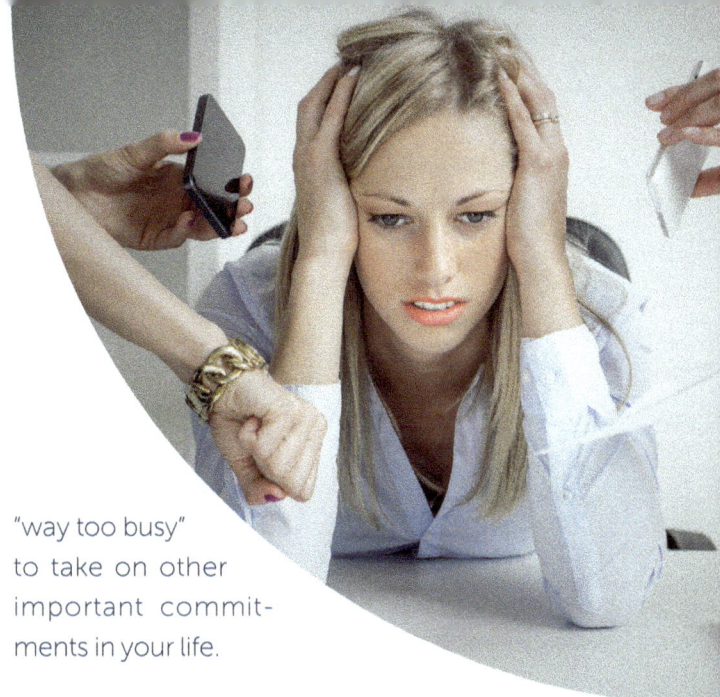

"way too busy" to take on other important commitments in your life.

Devote fifteen minutes a day to expanding your DRIVE profile ... do that consistently, day after day, as part of the holistic plan I am sharing with you in this book ... and you will tame your to-do list. That's a promise.

"I hate to work out."

There are a number of intriguing variations on this, including, "I guess I'm just too lazy," and, "That's not the kind of person I am." They're common excuses because others are unlikely to challenge them. But they need to be challenged.

Reality check: Nine times out of ten, when I hear this excuse, and I interact with the person who is using it, I find out that what they are really saying is, "I hate the way I have been working out up to this point." You're not lazy. You're not the "kind of" person who is designed not to move. (There is no such person.) You just haven't found a formula that works for you ... yet.

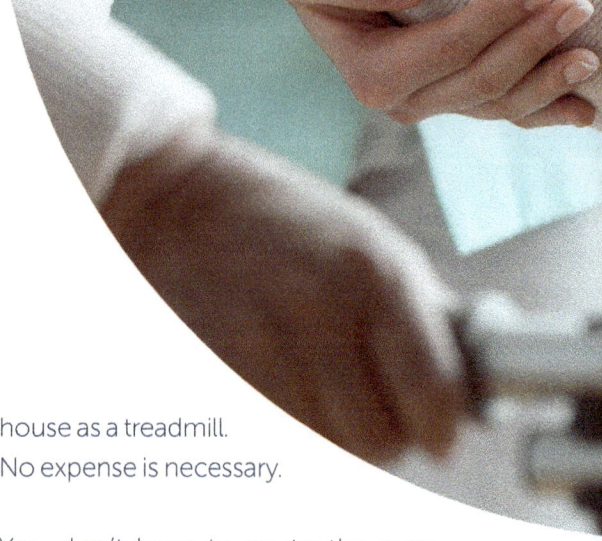

The simplest and most effective way to turn the limiting "I hate to work out" belief around is to follow the advice I've shared with you elsewhere in this book: *take action with your Accountability Partner.* Make this a social activity and build some mutual commitment into it. In almost every case I have seen, this takes an activity that the person "hated" and turns it into something to look forward to. There are any number of great ways to do this, including joining a gym together, taking a walk together, or (my favorite) building a comprehensive, escalating plan together, using the GOOD/BETTER/BEST activities you'll find at the end of this chapter.

When in doubt ... get a buddy involved! Set some goals and execute those goals together.

"I can't afford it."

I'm always surprised at how often this one comes up. It doesn't bear any scrutiny at all. I think of it as the "I can't come up with any other reason" excuse.

Reality Check: No one is saying you have to join a gym. No one is saying you have to buy any fancy gizmos or equipment. No one is saying you have to get a whole new workout wardrobe. If you *want* to do any of those things, that's fine. But they are absolutely not required.

What is required? You. A specific daily time commitment. And your environment, whatever that may be. You can use the stairs in your home as a Stairmaster if you want. You can use the road outside your house as a treadmill. No expense is necessary.

You don't have to go to the gym or spend a lot of money on equipment to get healthier.

All you need is a willingness to go outside your comfort zone.

And guess what? Your comfort zone is the root of the problem!

All the excuses I've shared with you are all saying something else. They are all, when you get right down to it, reformulations of a universal, underlying excuse, one that people don't like to say out loud:

"I am too comfortable with what I am familiar with to make the effort to change."

At the base of all the objections is the fact that people have become comfortable with not moving. Here's the reality check on that one: *How much is your comfort costing you?*

Comfort breeds complacency. Complacency is expensive. Make sure you understand what you're

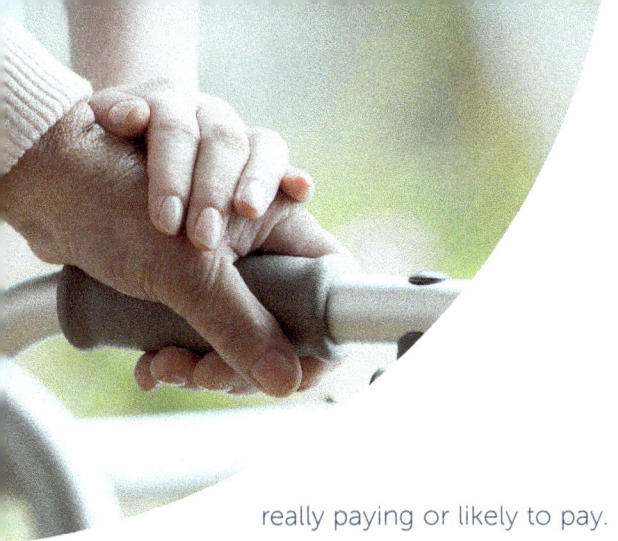

THE AGING MYTH

It's easy to fall into the pattern I described above. It's easy to stay in our comfort zones and avoid physical movement. But we have to challenge ourselves in this area because:

Not Moving Enough = Disaster

really paying or likely to pay. Don't become lazy!

A stressful, sedentary lifestyle – one where I didn't move very much during the course of the average day – was in my comfort zone for a good long stretch of my life. I've already shared with you what that got me: an agonizing case of kidney stones, a serious health crisis, and a lecture from my doctor that I was literally risking death if I didn't change the way I was living. I wrote this book so you could get out of your comfort zone before something similar happened in your life.

Complacency is not good in business. It destroys companies. It has no place in our personal lives or our health because it destroys our bodies just as predictably. Getting comfortable is a swindle. It's a lie we tell ourselves. Eventually, it leads you to the kind of severe discomfort you and your family definitely don't want.

> "All you need us a willingness to go outside your comfort zone."

You may think I'm exaggerating, but I can tell you from personal experience that it's no exaggeration. There's a cascading negative effect on our body, and it's not pretty. Lack of movement prevents waste products from being eliminated from the system, and if waste products don't get eliminated from the bloodstream, guess what happens? They get backed up. If waste products get backed up, nutrients won't get into our cells the way they should. Our muscles become weaker and smaller, and our joints will not be as strong as they should be. We won't have as much energy as we should. All those issues come together and worsen, eventually leading to a whole bunch of other problems and concerns that end up being misdiagnosed as part of this mysterious thing called *aging*.

Guess what? That's not *aging* at all. It's us neglecting our bodies and pumping our bloodstreams full of sewage. We see the consequences of that choice, and we think, "Oh, look at that, my body's having problems, I must be getting old." Wrong! I've studied enough centenarians – people who live to be over a hundred – to be able to tell you that the quality of people's lives does not automatically decline in this way when they hit 60, or 70, or

DRIVE

80 ... if they make a habit of *moving* and taking care of their body in the other important ways I've been sharing with you in this book. They don't have to deal with all those problems.

"You can live a 'youthful' lifestyle well into your 70s and 80s!"

Here's what I've learned about getting older. You don't have to accept kidney stones and lower stamina and joint problems. It doesn't have to be part of the way you age ... if you follow **LIVE-IT! 180°**, and specifically if you motivate yourself to keep moving. You can live a vigorous, joyous, "youthful" lifestyle well into your 70s and 80s! And why in the world wouldn't you?

I have grandchildren. That means I get to talk about this. Getting old doesn't have to mean arthritis, diabetes, aches and pains, and joint breakdown and knee replacement or any of the other physical ailments most people complain about and associate with "getting older."

Those problems are a function of us not sleeping right, not eating right, not moving enough, not connecting with others in a way that gives our life purpose and not handling our stress properly.

I used to be an old man. Now I'm not. I went through a period where I was having hip problems, and joint pains, and my knees were hurting. I had kidney stones. Old man stuff, right? Wrong!

LIVE-IT! 180° INSIGHT

Getting old does not have to mean aches and pains and disease. Those things are not synonymous with aging. Aging just means spending a longer period of time alive on the planet Earth. The big question is not how old you are, but whether you are choosing to follow a lifestyle that sedentary... or one that is active.

I wasn't moving enough. What I was eating was pretty good, but I was flunking out on the other parts of **LIVE-IT! 180°**, notably my movement routine. Then I changed all that, and I got my life back in balance again. So, guess what? Now I'm not an old man any more.

How does that Bob Dylan song go? "I was so much older then – I'm younger than that now."

Side note: One of the fascinating things you find when you study centenarians – people who live to be 100 years or older – is that, when they die, they typically don't die because of joint failure or arthritis, or kidney failure, or any other ailments we've been talking about. Wouldn't you expect them to die because of those issues if those issues were connected to the aging process? That's not what happens. If you take care of yourself properly in the years before you reach 100, your body just gets so old that it stops! I don't know about you … but that's how I want to go out, preferably while I'm sleeping.

Bottom line: However old you are, **movement is youth in action.** Movement can create a healthy structural stress on your body that strengthens your bones and muscles and can keep you younger, longer. Movement can circulate the lymph and cleans you out and makes you stronger, longer. Movement can make you happier, longer, too. If you're looking for the key to a younger lifestyle, here it is: Get out of your comfort zone, walk away from the television, and start moving more! If you think movement is boring, you're wrong. *Television* is boring in comparison with a hike or a night of bowling with someone you love. Try it! See for yourself!

THE ADVANTAGES OF MOVEMENT

Maybe you're wondering what a lot of people are wondering at this stage: Why make the effort to change? What's the reward for doing so? What are the advantages of getting out and moving more than you're moving right now?

Glad you asked. Let's take look at four big pluses.

First of all, by moving more, you will **improve your mental health.** You will be clearer and more focused, and you will have a sense of deeper well-being. This is because the right level of physical activity releases endorphins that give you a sense of calm and pleasure and relaxation, a natural high. Your body's Intelligent Design wants you to enjoy movement that accelerates your heart rate for a sustained period, and it wants you to do that more often.

A vigorous workout routine also **delays the aging process.** People feel younger and healthier. Whatever your age now, however sedentary you may be now, you can expect to experience more from life, and prolong optimum brain and body functioning, and get out and do more in your sixties, seventies, eighties, and beyond if you start upgrading your movement habits today. If that's not enough to motivate somebody, I don't know what is. Yes, the scientists have signed off on this. Take a look:

WANT YOUR BODY AND BRAIN TO LAST LONGER? MOVE!

"(A)Harvard study … found that previously sedentary men who began exercising after the age of 45 enjoyed a 24% lower death rate than their classmates who remained inactive. The maximum benefits were linked to an amount of exercise equivalent to walking for about 45 minutes a day at about 17 minutes per mile. On average, sedentary people gained about 1.6 years of life expectancy from becoming active later in life. Stud-

ies from Harvard, Norway, and England all confirm the benefits of exercise later in life. It's important research, but it confirms the wisdom of the Roman poet Cicero, who said, 'No one is so old that he does not think he could live another year.' "

https://www.health.harvard.edu/staying-healthy/exercise-and-aging-can-you-walk-away-from-father-time

"Telomeres are protective caps found at the ends of chromosomes that help keep them stable—not unlike how the plastic sheath at the end of shoelaces stops them from fraying. Every time a cell divides, telomeres get shorter. Eventually they become too small to protect the chromosomes and cells get old and die—resulting in aging. Shorter telomeres are related to many age-related diseases, including cancer, stroke and cardiovascular disease... Exercise science professor Larry Tucker from Brigham Young University compared telomere length with levels of physical activity. His findings showed significant differences between those who did regular, vigorous exercise and those who did not. "Just because you're 40, doesn't mean you're 40 years old biologically," he said in a statement. "We all know people that seem younger than their actual age. The more physically active we are, the less biological aging takes place in our bodies." He discovered adults with a high level of physical activity had a "biological aging advantage" of nine years compared to sedentary adults. When compared with those who did a moderate amount of exercise, the difference for highly active adults was seven years... "Overall, physical activity was significantly and meaningfully associated with telomere length in U.S. men and women," he wrote. "Evidently, adults who participate in high levels of physical activity tend to have longer telomeres, accounting for years of reduced cellular aging compared to their more sedentary counterparts."

http://www.newsweek.com/exercise-anti-aging-younger-cellular-level-telomeres-607228

"Physical activity can slow brain aging by as much as 10 years, reports a new study published in the journal Neurology. It's among the first studies to actually put a number on how beneficial exercise can be for the brain. The researchers asked a group of 1,228 men and women of diverse racial and ethnic backgrounds living in Manhattan about their regular exercise habits. They also answered questions that tested their cognitive abilities, including their memory, organization, reasoning and thinking speed. Five years later, they performed the same tests on about half of the study group. People who reported doing more physical activity showed higher scores on cognitive tests—consistent with previous studies linking more exercise to better brain health."

http://time.com/4269672/exercise-brain-aging/

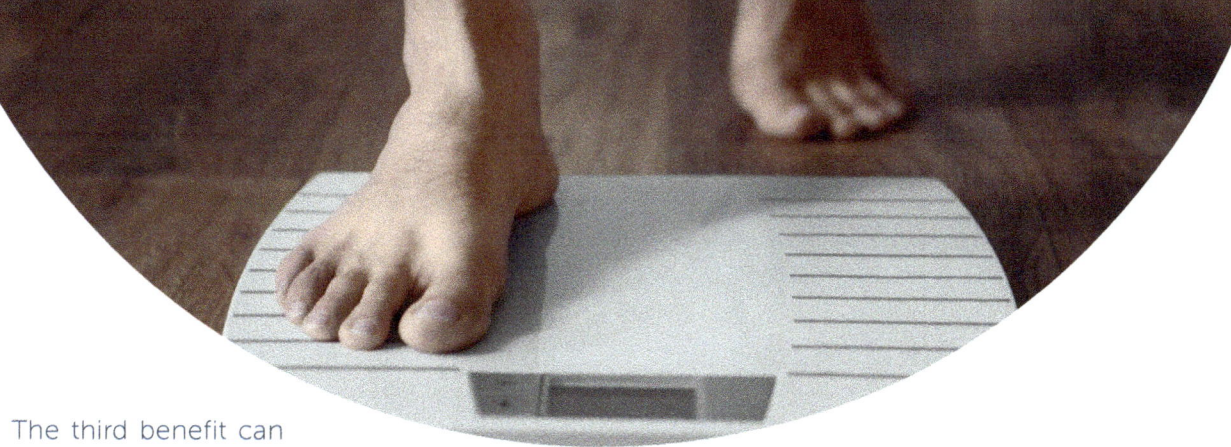

The third benefit can be a bigger motivator for some people than either of the other two: **weight loss**. I think this is because obesity carries a such significant social impact. Whatever motivates you works for me!

Reduced weight is indeed one of the huge advantages that many people experience from accelerating their workout routine. It's simple math, really. A good workout session helps you lose weight by burning more calories than you're taking in. When that happens, you burn fat and start losing weight. In fact, if you're taking in all the nutrients you need and following the FUEL guidelines I shared with you in a previous chapter, the only thing you're going to lose by upping your workout routine is fat. And when you've got enough muscle built up in your body, guess what? You're even going to burn fat while you sleep.

A side note: Some people who dramatically ramp up their movement routine build up a lot of muscle at the same time that they burn off fat. This can lead to a situation where the weight loss is minimal or nonexistent ... for the simple reason that muscle weighs more than fat! What's important to notice in this situation is that your body-mass index is headed in the right direction. The muscle to fat ratio is improving ... and that's a good thing! You are happier and healthier, and that's what counts.

Last, but not least: Improving your movement routine **strengthens your heart and lungs**. This means that your body circulates oxygen and nutrients more effectively ... and you give yourself a stronger foundation for good health and a vibrant sense of well-being in countless other areas. Improved heart and lung function have been linked to increased HDL (good) blood cholesterol level, reduced risk of diabetes and hypertension, stronger bones, and a lower risk of stroke.

MUSCLE PLIABILITY

A six-year-old takes a bad fall off a bike and bounces right back, with lots of crying but no major injury. A *forty*-six-year old takes a fall off a bike and may not cry ... but sustains major muscle and tendon damage. What's the big difference? Is it possible the kid's muscles and tendons are in better shape than the grownups?

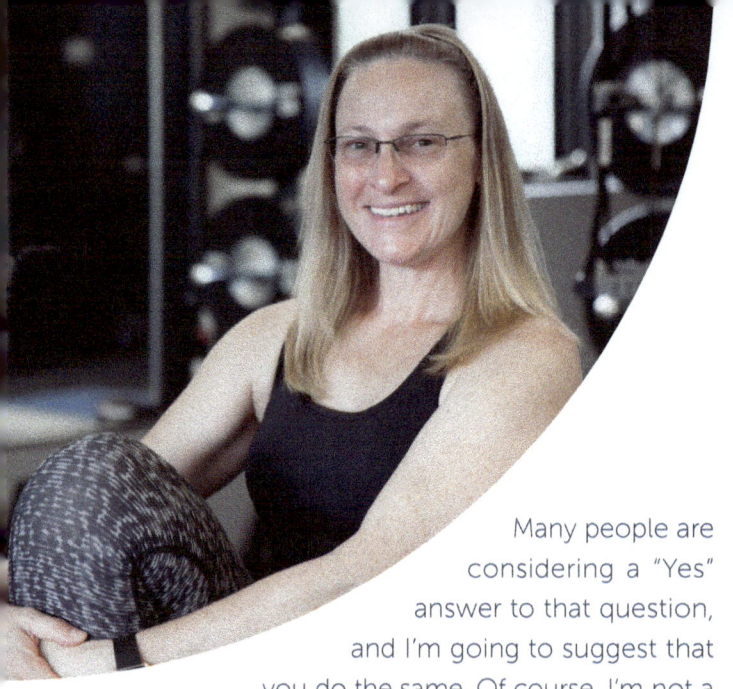

Many people are considering a "Yes" answer to that question, and I'm going to suggest that you do the same. Of course, I'm not a doctor, so I can't tell you what the perfect exercise routine is for you. What I can do, though, is share a critical *training principle* that I've been practicing in my own workouts and with the people I coach, since 1987, which I've found to be extremely effective for all age groups and fitness levels. This principle is known as *muscle pliability*. It's built around the idea of getting our muscles back to the optimum state we enjoyed when we were six, seven, or eight years old – before we twisted them up and made them less pliable than they were designed to be. This is all too easy to do, by the way. It's roughly the equivalent of letting the tires on your car become underinflated and out of alignment ... and then letting them stay underinflated and out of alignment for ten or fifteen years. The car's performance is going to suffer, as does your body when your muscles lose their pliability. An exercise routine that restores their youthful pliability gets everything back into the manufacturer's recommended operating range.

Truth be told, I am pretty sure I *came up* with this idea as a conditioning method back in the late Eighties. It's all over the place now, having been prominently embraced by the NFL quarterback Tom Brady, who credits muscle pliability with extending his remarkable career. I choose to take that as high praise, though Tom has yet to drop me a thank-you note. (I guess he's been busy.) On the other side of the argument, though, is the reality that principles behind the workout approach we now call muscle pliability have deep roots in Eastern medicine. For all I know the techniques may have been in play in the Orient for centuries.

This may be one of those great ideas that has a hundred or more different "originators." What I am confident of, though, is that no one I ran into in the United States was doing this before I started doing it ... and I talked to a lot of people. At the end of the day, though, who gets credit for this really doesn't matter. What matters is that people use it.

By this point, I bet you're wondering: What exactly, is muscle pliability? Fortunately, there is a simple answer. It's a conditioning strategy that results in the lengthening of muscles that are under duress. This conditioning process, which incorporates massage while the trainee is moving and contracting a specific muscle, breaks down and flushes out adhesions, scar tissue, congestion, and knotting – all of which are sources of major distress to the body. The idea is to force out stress and toxins and lengthen the muscle to its optimum size.

The key word here is "optimum." Traditional strength training has, for decades, focused on lifting heavy weights and de-emphasized or ignored the slow, careful lowering of that weight. The result is that muscles are "developed" in a way that stresses the body and shortens the muscle in question.

That's a problem, because each muscle has an optimum size, just like every tire has an optimum inflation pressure. If a muscle is too short, you can only produce force in very limited ranges of motion, and it applies stress to the joints that are attached. The problem isn't muscles that are long and relaxed. The problem is muscles that are too short and overstressed. That Popeye-cartoon image of the muscle popping up like a little hill from your bicep turns out to be the exact opposite of what we should all be after – although a lot of workout coaches have yet to figure this out.

Make no mistake: You will need the help of a qualified conditioning coach to enjoy the full benefits of a routine that incorporates the muscle pliability approach: forcing out stress and toxins, and improving recovery times and longevity, by lengthening the distressed muscle. Feel free to reach out to us at coachpete@liveit180.com if you need help finding a coach. You can also visit LiveIt180.com! In the meantime, consider the following possibilities:

- Work out with lower-resistance (that is, lighter) weights. If world class professional athletes don't need heavy barbells, maybe you don't, either.

- Take at least as much time releasing the weight as you do raising it. The big idea here is balance.

- Choose range-of-motion exercises that move your joints through their full trajectory ... rather than narrower, high-pressure, high-stress exercises that push muscles and tendons to the absolute limit of their capacity within just a portion of the joint's arc.

- Use foam rolling, deep tissue neuromuscular massage, stretch bands, and active range of motion techniques with a qualified practitioner.

GOOD, BETTER, **BEST**: PERSONALIZE LIVE-IT! 180°

There are as many good approaches to the DRIVE principle as there are people reading this book. Even so, you can break down the way you choose to take action on this principle into three broad categories. The system is designed to maximize your options and give you flexibility to get MOVING in the way that feels best to you.

Important: Before you embark on any exercise routine – including but not limited to any of the ideas you'll find below – be sure to consult with your personal physician.

Here's how it breaks down.

"GOOD" – PHASE ONE

- First and foremost, understand that this phase is all about meeting you where you are. If you've been following the plan thus far, you're already doing some basic DRIVE activity by taking a walk for between fifteen and thirty minutes a day. This is the foundation of all the suggestions that follow – so please keep that up.

- In addition, at the GOOD level, I'm going to encourage you to identify at least one other element of movement that you personally enjoy doing and to do that for an additional five to ten minutes a day, on top of the daily walk you're used to. This is really up to you. It could be five more minutes of walking, it could be doing jumping jacks with your spouse or significant other, it could be jogging, it could be getting on the Stairmaster – it's your call. Whatever it is, just make sure you love it. Once you've done that and feel comfortable with it...

- Set up a targeted weekly workout routine, ideally in a group at a local fitness center, but that part is up to you. Here at the top tier of the GOOD phase, your week should, in addition to the two items listed above, look like this:

   » Mondays and Thursdays: Do a whole-body workout for 30 minutes. That workout should begin with something like running in place or doing jumping jacks, an activity that gets your heart rate up, and should then move on to *pulling, pushing, bending, squatting,* and *working on your core* movements. Close the session out with another exercise that gets your heart pumping.

» Tuesdays and Friday: Straight cardio blast for thirty minutes. This means half an hour of something that gets your heart pumping – for instance, jogging or swimming.
» Wednesdays and Saturdays: Stretching and breathing for thirty minutes. This means stretching every major part of your body, starting with your neck and working your way down to your shoulders, arms, elbows, wrists, back, stomach, hips, legs, thighs, and hamstrings. Repeat the cycle. Don't hurt yourself. Stretch in a way you are comfortable with for the first twenty to twenty-five minutes; relax and breathe for the final five to ten minutes.
» Sunday: This is your day off. Take a break.

IMPORTANT: This schedule is expressly designed to give your body a break and allow it to restore itself between the different movement cycles. There is no religious significance to having Sunday as your day off; you can feel free to move the days forward or backward, but keep the same calendar intervals between exercise types.

You can stop there or move on to ...

"BETTER" – PHASE TWO:

Do everything in the "GOOD" phase – but alter your targeted workout routine in the following important way:

- *Start using weights during your whole-body workout days.* It's best to start small. Just make sure you use some kind of weight to focus on each of your body's major muscle groups. Cover all the groups during each thirty-minute session.

If you get comfortable with this level and find you want to move on to the next phase, good for you! That would be...

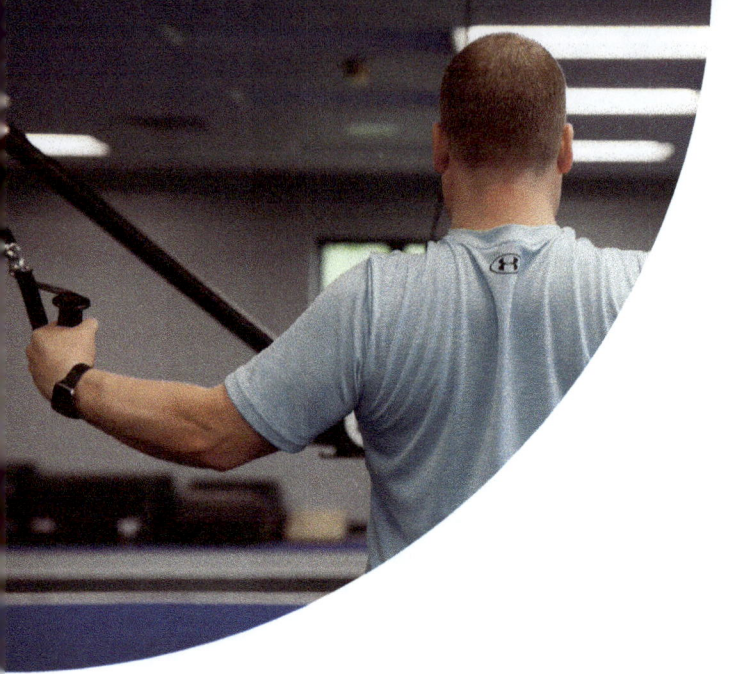

THE LIVE-IT! 180° WEBSITE

In addition to the previous suggestions for setting up a personalized Good, Better, and Best approach to DRIVE, I've added a lot of additional material on our website, LiveIt180.com, that will help you to make the principle fun and challenging. There you'll find a DRIVE challenge you can sign up for that will help you design, outline, and execute your perfect workout – and give you challenges and encouragements that will coach you for up to a full year of activity. Check it out!

Earlier in this chapter, I discussed how important it is to take control of the mental aspect of your workout routine. Let me remind you once again, before we move on to CONNECT, that what you've read here is an important resource that will help you to keep your head in the right place when it comes to working out regularly. Return to this part of the book often and reread it as necessary. If you find yourself plateaued or not moving at all, use this chapter to reignite your passion and motivate you to DRIVE!

"BEST" – PHASE THREE

This is just like the "BETTER" phase, with the following important exception: You will now work with a qualified fitness coach on Mondays and Thursdays to do the focused, "chiseling" work. This is a professional-grade workout that uses advanced techniques to get you to a point where you have a specific physique that you choose. Here, you are using weight training with precision to develop specific opposing muscle groups. Although it's wonderful if you get to this point, there is absolutely nothing wrong with *not* reaching this level.

A FINAL THOUGHT

I've laid out a flexible, but powerful, workout routine for you – but remember that the most important part of the DRIVE principle is simply taking *some* kind of physical action to get your heart pumping and place good stress on your muscles. Some people can do a weekly workout

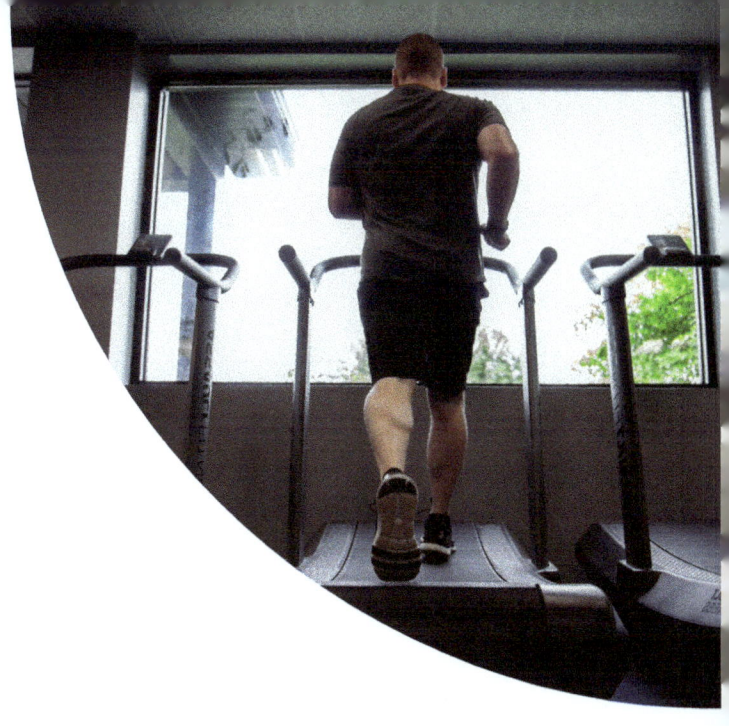

routine like the one I've outlined here, and some people can't. The right plan is *your* plan. If you and your doctor decide that the low end of the "GOOD" phase – just taking a walk once a day – is right for you, then go for it. If that's where you find yourself, though, my challenge to you is a simple one: Find a way to rock that walk, each and every day … and see how you can build on it. At every phase, **LIVE-IT! 180°** takes you on from wherever you are right now, and that's particularly true about the DRIVE principle.

At *any given moment, you have the choice between moving and doing nothing … so get out there and DRIVE!* Make the most of where you are right now and grow from there.

> *"All truly great thoughts are conceived while walking."*
>
> —Friedrich Nietzsche, Twilight of the Idols

Plan your life and live your plan. LIVE-IT! 180°!

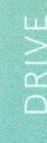

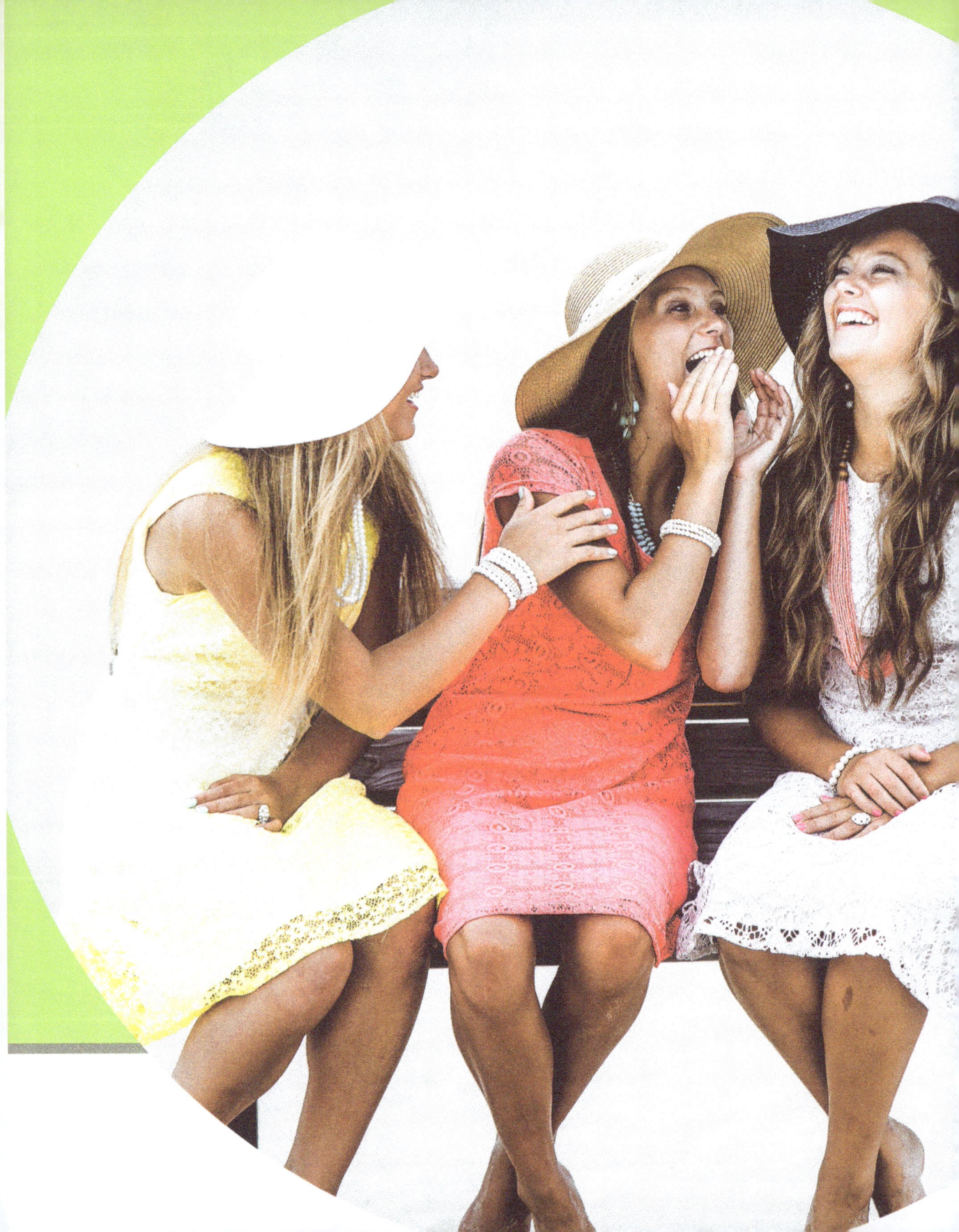

CONNECT

Set your personal destination by building a sense of purpose and social interaction into your daily life.

8

Set your destination ... by building a sense of purpose and social interaction into your daily life.

We now move from DRIVE to CONNECT.

In earlier chapters, I suggested that you think of sleep as the battery that starts your car and consider food as the fuel for that superior, Intelligently Designed vehicle. Then in the DRIVE chapter, I asked you to take that car out for a spin on a regular basis – to remember that leaving it undriven for long periods of time is asking for trouble. Now, in this chapter, I want to ask you this simple question: *Where are you going in that car? What's your destination? What's your purpose?*

Every good journey has a destination – and in the journey of life, our intended destination is the same thing as our *purpose*. We're human beings, which means that our purpose involves *other* human beings. We weren't designed to operate solo. We're designed to have a destination that matters not only to us, but to others. Just like a car connects with a satellite signal to activate its navigation system and identify its destination, we need to CONNECT with other human beings and build a sense of direction, a sense of purpose in our lives ... every day.

That's what this principle is all about – interacting with other people. Feeling needed. Being a part of a family or tribe. Getting out there. Adding something to someone else's day. In person. In other words, getting, being, and staying CONNECTED!

Some people are surprised that this should be part of a so-called "fitness" program. Actually, it makes perfect sense to give CONNECT this kind of emphasis. If you want a healthy lifestyle, you want things to be in balance in your life. This means that as well as sleeping right, eating right, and working out, you need to have good social and family relationships. If these relationships aren't in place, there's no way to be in a state of vibrant health. *We are tribal beings – happy, healthy human beings do not exist independent of the tribe.*

That tribe may be a knitting club, a sales team, the 82nd Airborne Division, or something else. One thing the tribe *isn't*, though, is Facebook and Twitter and Instagram. I'm not saying you have to give those things up – just that you shouldn't mistake them for CONNECT!

Thanks to Intelligent Design, we thrive by means of *face-to-face* interactions with other people. All of us have room for improvement in this area. In this chapter, you'll learn how to maximize and improve those interactions. Just like the other parts of **LIVE-IT! 180°**, CONNECT is not just a suggestion. CONNECT is critical to losing weight, living fit, and enjoying life!

WHY BOTHER WITH THIS?

You may not be used to thinking of your social life as integral to your health and well-being. As a matter of fact, you're probably a little surprised that this chapter even exists. You may even be wondering how big an impact something like connecting with other people could have on your overall quality of life.

It's natural for people to feel that way, and in a way, I'm glad this skepticism exists. Why? Because most of us assume that our ability to connect with others is something that more or less takes care of itself, and that whether or not we aim to make changes in this area of our life, the impacts on our overall quality of life are minimal. We are far more likely to focus on making lifestyle changes that affect our weight and our level of physical activity than we are to make changes that affect our level of interaction with others.

That's a big mistake.

The scientific evidence is in on this, and the results are clear. People who aren't good at making and sustaining connections with others *die a whole lot sooner* than people who are good at making and sustaining connections with others. That's the bottom line: *Not connecting means you don't live as long.* Consider the following:

> • A comprehensive study of 7,000 men and women in California found that people who were "disconnected from others" were "roughly three times more likely to die during the nine-year study than people with strong social ties."

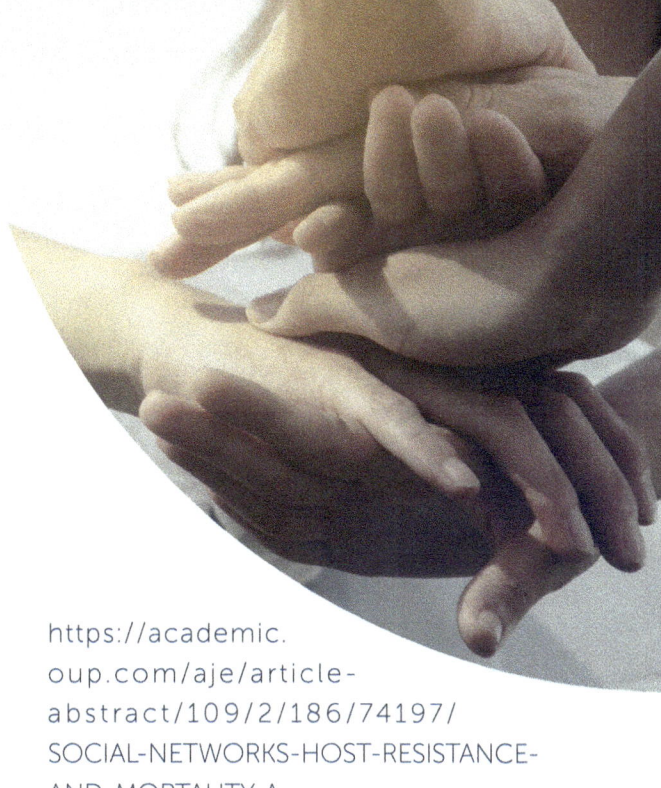

https://academic.oup.com/aje/article-abstract/109/2/186/74197/SOCIAL-NETWORKS-HOST-RESISTANCE-AND-MORTALITY-A

• A similarly rigorous study involving 6,500 people in England found that "limited contact with family, friends, and community groups predicts illness and earlier death, regardless of whether it is accompanied by feelings of loneliness." http://www.nature.com/news/social-isolation-shortens-lifespan-1.12673

• A study of over 2,000 men in New York who had suffered heart attacks found that those with "strong connections to other people" had only 25% of the risk of death in the three years following their attack than men who were socially isolated. http://www.nejm.org/doi/pdf/10.1056/NEJM198408303110902

- An analysis of existing research on the link between social interaction and longevity carried out by Brigham Young University found that "having social ties with friends, family, neighbors, and colleagues can improve our odds of survival by 50 percent." Researchers also found that behavior that neglected such ties, meaning long-term behavior leading to "low social interaction," had "a similar impact on lifespan as being an alcoholic or smoking 15 cigarettes a day." This behavior, the researchers concluded, was more harmful than physical inactivity, and twice as harmful as obesity. https://www.medicalnewstoday.com/articles/196056.php

LIVE-IT! 180° TIP

Get face-to-face. Get personal. Get connected. Social isolation is a silent, insidious killer! Overcoming it means turning off your phone, turning off your TV, turning off your computer, and making a real-time connection with one or more human beings who are literally present in your physical environment.

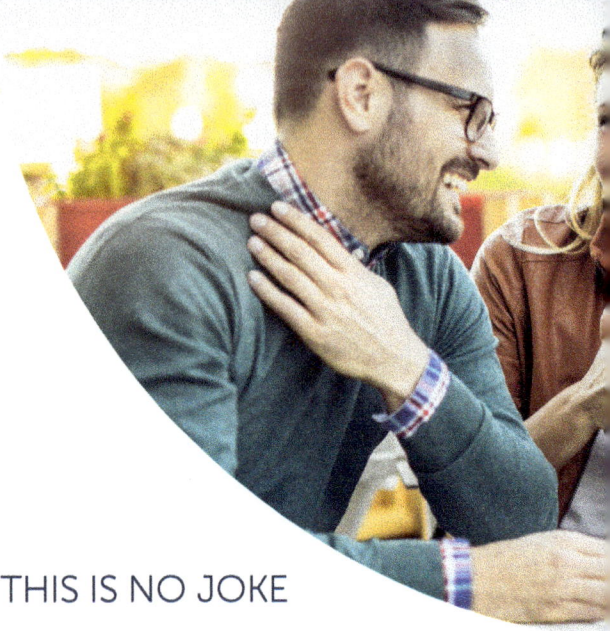

THIS IS NO JOKE

I could go on, but I think you get the idea. In a period of human history when we're relying more and more on digital interactions with people we can't see and less and less on face to face interactions with people we can, underestimating the importance of making connections with others is a potentially huge problem. And it's one we all need to pay attention to.

At this point, I'm going to share something with you that the research studies do *not* seem to have pointed out. I don't have hard data to back it up, but I know for a fact that this is true, from personal experience and from interactions with the many people I've coached over the years: *It's all connected ... and we ignore that at our peril.* Simply focusing on *one* of these issues is a major part of the problem. We should *notice* when the scientists tell us that a lack of social activity is as dangerous as alcohol or cigarettes, potentially more dangerous to us than physical inactivity or obesity. But...

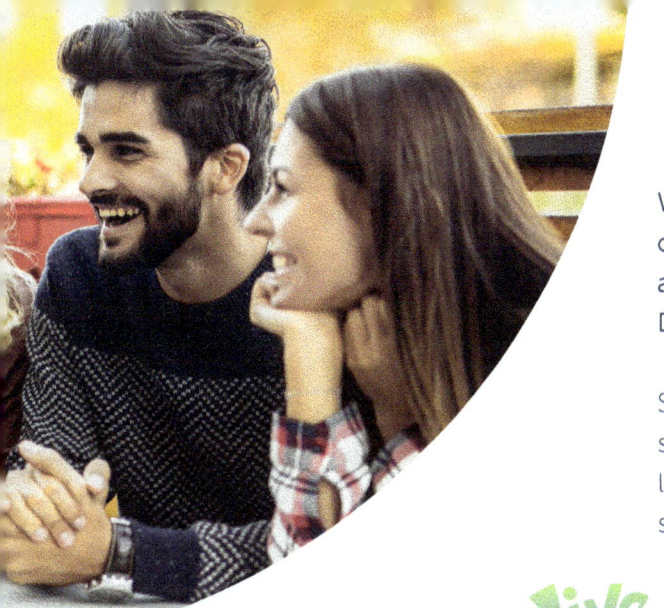

What we *really* need to notice is that we reduce our lifespan and our quality of life whenever we are out of *balance* with the way our Intelligent Design intended us to live.

So: making an in-person connection and in-person contributions to the community in which we live is part of maintaining that balance, just like sleep, just like eating right, just like movement,

LIVE-IT! 180° INSIGHT

What's the very worst punishment the criminal justice system can come up with? I'll give you a hint. It's not the death penalty. Many experts in the field believe that a lifetime of solitary confinement – the prospect of never speaking to anyone again for the rest of your life – is likelier to have a more powerful deterrent effect than execution. http://newsinfo.inquirer.net/793268/solitary-confinement-worse-than-death-zubiri

Even the most hardened, self-sufficient subjects melt into pools of psychosis and dysfunction when they are deprived of human contact. One 1951 study of extreme solitary confinement was designed to last six weeks – but had to be called off because none of the subjects could function beyond the six-day mark. *This is Mother Nature telling us something: Contact with other people is important to our health and wellbeing!*

Connect is just like Recharge, Fuel, and Drive – we need to get the right amount of human interaction every day. Specifically, we need to make a certain amount of *contribution* every day. Connection and *contribution* are really two sides of the same coin. Unfortunately, many of us in the modern, online, social-media-driven, "connected" world aren't getting our minimum daily requirements of either connection or contribution. For a people who are so connected, we are really not connected at all!

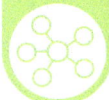

and just like repairing your "car" with preventive maintenance.

Bottom line: This is part of your owner's manual for your Intelligently Designed machine. If you want it to function at an optimum level, you need to find a way to up your game in the area of social connection! This is not an optional, "elective" choice. It's something that will literally add years to your life ... *if* you upgrade while you are building and reinforcing your LIVE-IT! 180° daily lifestyle.

A TRUE STORY ABOUT CONNECTION AND CONTRIBUTION

Here's something that really happened to someone I know. I'll call him Jake. Jake's story plays out in three phases.

PHASE ONE: Jake was working long hours at a job he wasn't crazy about – a job that he felt was keeping him from moving to the next phase of his personal development. He felt isolated and in a rut. One day, a friend approached him and made a point of spending some one-on-one time with him. During that one-on-one leisure time, the friend asked Jake a great question: *What do you really want to do with your life?*

Notice what happened in Phase One: Someone made an effort to spend quality one-on-one time with Jake. It didn't happen by accident. His buddy scheduled the time and showed up in person. Jake told his buddy what he wanted to do with his life and his career, to get into sales and marketing.

PHASE TWO: Shortly after this, something remarkable happened. As it happened, Jake's buddy was looking for qualified salespeople. By "qualified," Jake's buddy really meant two things: motivated and willing to learn. He wasn't all that concerned with the level of professional experience Jake brought to the table. What he was interested in was the commitment to produce results. Deciding that Jake had that commitment, the buddy offered Jake a job as a salesperson. Jake accepted. Here's the cool part: Within three years, Jake had worked his way up to a senior executive position at his buddy's company.

Now notice what really took place in Phase Two: Jake found a *tribe* he could contribute to, and he started pushing himself out of his comfort zone in order to be able to *make* that contribution. He started to look past his old horizons. He started to learn and grow. (That's the cool thing about being part of a tribe – you get to develop your competencies and expand the scale at which you contribute.)

PHASE THREE: Three years on, Jake is now one of the key people at his buddy's

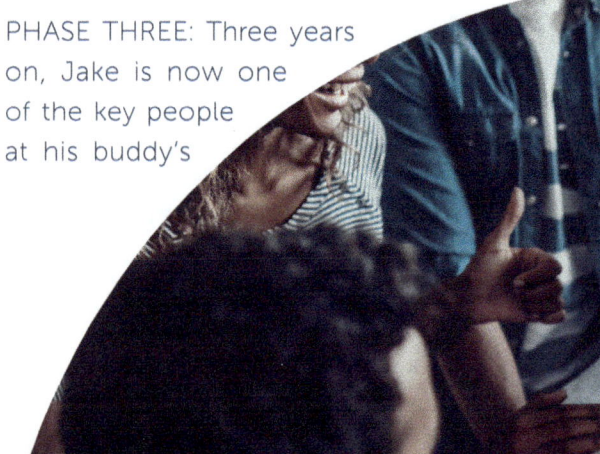

company ... and he's not only contributing professionally, he's active as *part of the team* in about a half-dozen charitable pursuits the company sponsors, notably a mission to help the homeless. Jake goes out there with the rest of the team on a regular basis, helping as part of a company effort designed to give something back to the community.

Here's what I want you to notice about Phase Three: Jake is now taking part in a series of *organized social events* based on the idea of contributing as a tribe. This is social connection with the specific aim of making a difference. It involves helping a person or group of people without any expectation of payment or material gain.

Look at the sequence again:

Phase One: Connect one-on-one with someone in your world.

Phase Two: Connect with a tribe and contribute to that tribe.

Phase Three: Take part in a charitable social activity your tribe commits to as a group.

Notice that there is a progression here from the one-on-one connection, to the connection of the individual to the tribe, and finally to the connection of the tribe to the larger human community. This progression is deeply ingrained in the Intelligently Designed machine that is the human body. It's part of our wiring. It's how we are designed to operate. And finding a tribe you can be part of – not just digitally, not just virtually, but in person and in real time – is central to the experience of being human. This can literally be a life-saving experience. Finding the purpose and meaning of YOUR life is critical to living healthy, happier, and younger. If you want to lose weight, live fit, and enjoy life, being connected is critical. People need people, and we all need to find our purpose and pursue it.

By the way, I'm using the word "tribe" here to mean **a group of people who interact with each other and are dependent on each other.** You don't have to look very hard to figure out that human beings are designed to be interdependent, and that they are meant to function in groups that make life easier and more connected for each member of the group than it would be if they each tried to go it alone. A tribe could also be a neighborhood or your own personal family, where people look out for each other. You can get a clear sense of just how important such social gatherings are if you take a look at the Okinawa culture in Japan.

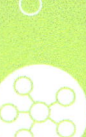

CLOSE UP ON THE OKINAWA CULTURE

The Okinawa prefecture, an island group in Japan, is noted for something that should be of interest to every reader of this book: the longevity and vibrant health of its people.

Research has confirmed that Okinawans not only have the longest life expectancy in the world, they also have the longest *health* expectancy, meaning their high quality of life is derived not just from living longer but from living longer without debilitating disease. Japanese government statistics confirm that there are 34.7 centenarians for every 100,000 Okinawans – easily the highest mark yet measured in any community in the world. Research also confirms that these people have significantly lower rates of cancer, heart attack, Alzheimer's disease, and stroke than other groups. They also report many people in their nineties with active, satisfying sex lives.

The obvious question is: Why? What makes Okinawans live so long – and age so slowly? And here's my answer: Broadly speaking, these people are following the main aspects of **LIVE-IT! 180°**. Specifically, their lifestyle is notable for its low-carb diet that includes vegetables/fruits/nuts/fish/healthy fats, for good sleep routines, for emphasizing physical activity, and for a tradition of social connection and a deep sense of personal purpose arising from contribution to community. These factors all play a huge role in their longevity, as does a cultural emphasis on effective stress reduction via outlets such as meditation.

In the Okinawan islands, there is a concept known as "Yuima-ru," which translates as "the circle of the people." In essence, it means taking care of each other, throughout the entire course of the human life cycle. Community ties are extremely strong in Okinawa, and supportive interaction within groups, clubs, and other social units is a long-standing tradition.

Just as important is the concept of "Ikigai," or purpose – one's personal reason for getting up in the morning. This is a hallmark of community and personal life in Okinawa, and just about everyone in an Okinawan community not only has such a reason for getting up but enjoys talking about it with others. One's Ikigai is not based on the amount of money one makes, or even on one's current circumstances, but rather on *what one is giving back to one's chosen tribe and to the larger community.* Here is a story from Okinawa that illustrates the principle perfectly:

As an Osaka woman lay in a deep coma, she suddenly had a vision: she was being taken up to heaven. There, she stood before the Voice of her ancestors.

The Voice asked, "Who are you?"

She replied, "I am the mayor's wife."

The Voice said, "I didn't ask you whose wife you were. I asked who YOU are."

The woman said, "I am the mother of five children."

The Voice replied, "I didn't ask whose mother you are. I asked who YOU are."

The woman said, "I am a schoolteacher."

The Voice said, "I didn't ask about your profession. I asked who YOU are."

The conversation went on like this for some time. Every answer the woman gave, the Voice rejected. Finally, she said, "I am the one who wakes up each morning to care for my family and to nurture the young minds of the children who attend my school."

The Voice made no reply to this. She was sent back to earth, where she emerged from her coma and woke each day at sunrise with a deep sense of meaning and purpose.

The woman in the story found her Ikigai.

Interestingly, one of the issues scientists have tried to isolate was whether the astonishing longevity numbers in Okinawa could be explained solely on the basis of genetics. The current thinking is this is *not* what's driving these figures – a huge exodus from Okinawa to Brazil has given scientists the chance to study a group with strong genetic commonality to the people in Okinawa, but no adherence to the diet, exercise, and social customs of their relatives in Japan. The Brazilian Okinawans have a life span nearly twenty years *shorter*. Here's the lesson I take away from that: Find your Ikigai! And follow **LIVE-IT! 180°**.

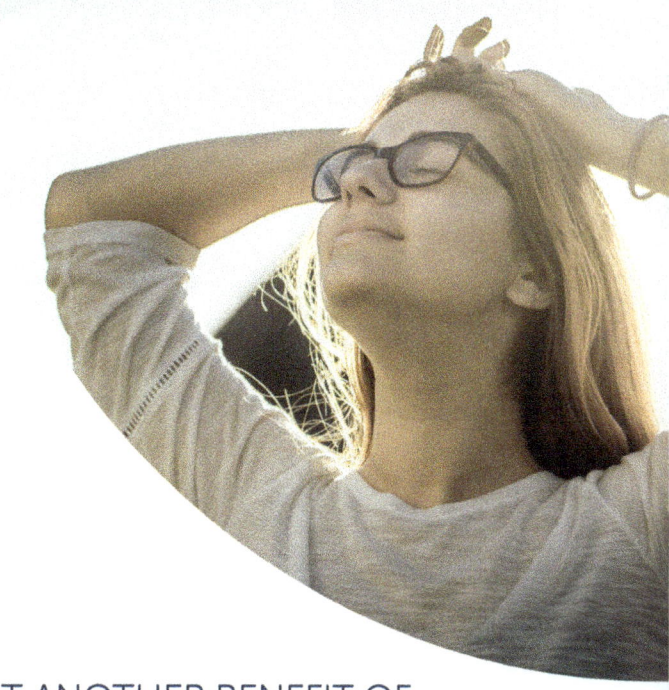

YET ANOTHER BENEFIT OF CONNECTING

Before I close this chapter, I have to share some important information with you that I haven't discussed yet. Now, this is something truly astonishing, something about that amazing, Intelligently Designed machine that is YOU that may seem counterintuitive at first but that really isn't. Please keep an open mind. Here it is:

You are designed to experience stress … and you're not functioning properly UNLESS you have the experience of stress.

Now, given what you may have heard elsewhere about the vital importance of "stress reduction" or "stress management," you're probably wondering if I've gone too far. You may even be thinking to yourself, "I've followed you through a lot of unlikely ideas, taken on a lot of new concepts that have pushed me out of my comfort zone, and done a

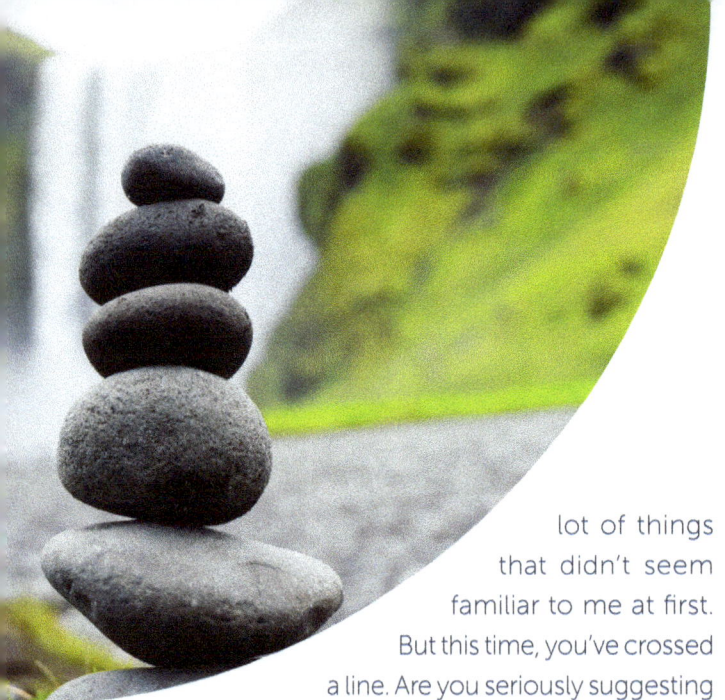

lot of things that didn't seem familiar to me at first. But this time, you've crossed a line. Are you seriously suggesting that respected doctors, researchers, and public health officials are going to tell me that stress is actually good for me?"

And the surprising answer to that question is: YES.

To understand how that could be so and how it connects to the **LIVE-IT! 180°** principle of CONNECT, you need to understand that modern medicine – following the groundbreaking work in the 1960s of a psychologist with the intriguing name of Richard Lazarus – has identified two *very different kinds of stress*: negative and positive.

The negative variety of stress, the kind we associate with poor health outcomes and shorter life spans, is technically known as *distress*. That label probably doesn't come as much of a surprise. Most of us are already familiar with the concept of distress, and it makes sense that being distressed on a regular basis is unlikely to be good for us.

What we may not be used to, though, and what may take a little more time to get our heads around, is the reality that there is flip-side to the stress coin, a side that's just as important for us to know about. The other side of that coin is called *eustress*, and it's the stress we experience that helps human beings to grow, expand, and achieve at an optimum level – to move beyond the comfort zone. It turns out that eustress is an important part of a healthy lifestyle – and an important part of social functioning.

To oversimplify, but not by much, eustress is the stress that you're *supposed* to experience on a regular basis – and much of it happens within the context of your relationships and connections with other people.

Eustress literally means "beneficial stress." This Greek/English hybrid word was coined by the endocrinologist Hans Selya. The term applies to psychological, physical, or biochemical stresses that elicit a positive response and deliver a positive health outcome. Notice that the psychological, physical, and biochemical responses *overlap*, because the human body operates in all three realms simultaneously. A psychological response affects your physical response and your biochemical response. There are wonderful hormones that are released during the eustress activity of sex for example. These hormones can lower blood pressure, calm the mind, and provide a sense of peace, a feeling of being wanted and loved, among many other benefits. All this comes from the positive stress placed on the body from having sex with your partner.

Other ways you can experiencing *eustress* include those situations when ...

- You're motivated in the face of a challenge

- You can feel yourself focusing your energy

- You perceive the stressful event as short-term as opposed to unending or lifelong

- You perceive the stressful event as being within your coping abilities

- You are excited

- Your performance improves

Can you think of an event that met all those criteria that happened to you within the last, say, 30 days? I'll bet you can. And guess what? Whatever it is for you, and whoever else it touched, you need that kind of stress on a regular basis, the same way you *need* air or water or sleep. It gives you a feeling of fulfilment. And your life really isn't complete without it.

So, let's review. You know there are not one, but *two* major types of stress – *distress and eustress,* or "bad stress" and "good stress." And you know that not all stress is bad. In fact, the "good stress" is essential to your well-being, because human beings are "wired" to experience this kind of stress and to use it to grow, achieve, and develop.

I'll deal with the topic of *distress* in much more detail in the next chapter. For now, though, what I want you to understand is that *eustress*, "good stress," often correlates to the quality of your relationships with other people.

You might experience it, for instance, as a result of getting a good grade on a test in a subject you thought was difficult, but your teacher thought you could handle. The exhilaration and fulfilment that comes from attaining an important goal is often rooted in some kind of interaction with another human being. Eustress is part of that. Obviously, your relationship with your teacher is going to affect the quality of your experience as you study for that test, and by the same token, your family relationships are going to affect the emotional and logistical support you get as you prepare for that test.

The stronger our relationships with other human beings, and the better our connections with them, the more fulfilling our eustress levels are going to be. The more disconnected we are from individuals, from our tribe, and from our larger community, the *less* of this essential stress we're going to experience. If you think you're going to catch up on your daily eustress requirement by playing video games with strangers you never meet in person, or reading novels, or engaging in any other essentially solitary activity ... you're wrong!

It's important to note that this is part of a much larger pattern, and that eustress goes beyond social connection. In our bodies, there are always good

stresses and bad stresses at work. For instance, let's say you're cooking something on the stove, and by mistake, you poke your finger into the path of the gas flame. What happens? You pull your finger back, of course. There's a stress response from your body that pulled your finger back automatically – in order to protect you. These kinds of stresses play out in our body all the time. It's a question of balancing them out.

Physical, mental, and structural stresses are always attacking the body, with the potential for causing damage and weakening our body's systems, particularly our immune systems. Fortunately, the counter-stress – eustress – can be brought to bear to heal the body and bring you back into the balance with your inner conductor, as our Intelligent Design intended.

As I promised, we'll take a much closer look at the other side of the stress "coin" in the next chapter of this book.

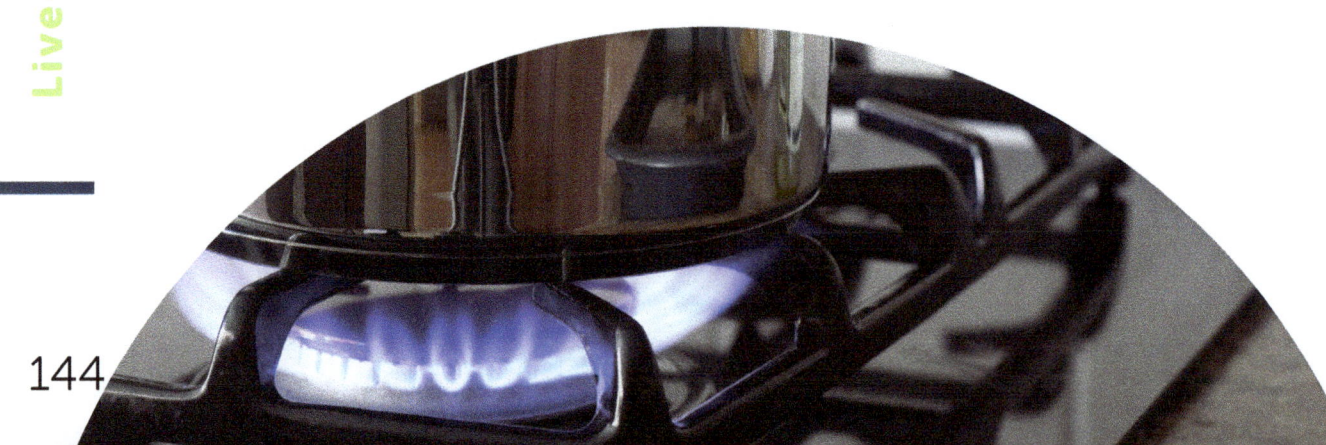

GOOD, BETTER, **BEST**: PERSONALIZE LIVE-IT! 180°

When it comes to connecting with others, the natural progression from GOOD to BETTER to BEST is something you want to build on. You don't stop doing the GOOD connection once you move up to the BETTER level, and you don't stop doing GOOD and BETTER once you work your way up to BEST. Your aim is to gradually expand your capacity to connect with others and contribute as part of a balanced, healthy way of life – one that's driven by Ikigai, or purpose.

Here's how this breaks down.

"GOOD" – PHASE ONE

Connect one-on-one with someone in your world.

In this initial phase, you make a conscious effort to connect in real time, face-to-face, in person, with another human being for at least twenty minutes. Notice that I said, "in person." We've talked a lot about "ghost food" in the book. Taking care of business in the realm of CONNECT means learning to set aside "ghost connections" – which are typically social media, video games, television, Netflix, and so forth. Connecting with your "friends" by sharing and liking their posts, or by binge-watching TV programs and sharing comments about them, or by watching the ballgame, *does not count* as the "Good" phase. Those are ghost connections. They're like the smoke and mirrors and the hovering face of the Wizard in the movie THE WIZARD OF OZ. There's no one there! Please understand that there's nothing wrong with these activities in the abstract, as long as they're part of a life lived in balance. But when you can't stop them, and you notice that they're keeping you from forming real interpersonal connections, they're what's called an *addiction*, and they need to be dealt with as such.

Here's how you beat a social media, or any media, addiction: Reach out and connect with a real human being, in person. I recommend you complete this weekly "Good" phase by picking any *two* activities from the following list that you will commit to doing at least once a week, for twenty minutes each. That's at least forty minutes of person-to-person (or if you choose the next-to-last option, person-to-animal) time, each week. Once you've made your choices, share your commitment with your accountability partner, and then follow through. Note that these interactions need to be in person, not phone or text messaging.

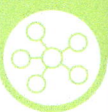

(Side note – you may already be doing these kinds of one-on-one, *in person* activities for sixty minutes a week as part of your personal routine. If that's the case – congratulations! Keep it up and move on to the BETTER phase.)

- Go for a walk with your spouse or significant other.

- Go for a walk with a friend or coworker.

- Go for a walk with a family member.

- Visit the gym with an exercise buddy.

- Reach out to someone at work you normally don't talk to and invite him or her out for a cup of coffee or tea.

- Visit a public place (like a cafe) and make a new friend.

- Visit a neighbor you know.

- Introduce yourself to a neighbor you *don't know* and invite him or her over to your place for coffee or tea. (It's never too late to do this!)

- Set up a networking meeting that supports your business/career goals. Again, make sure this happens face to face, not over the phone. (For instance: Ask your boss for advice on your career path within the company you work for, or if you're the boss, suggest a meeting to *offer* an employee advice and help on his or her career path.)

- Spend some quality time with a pet. (Don't laugh. This is a great option that I can't recommend highly enough. Interacting with a pet gives you a sense of calm, lowers your blood pressure, and gives you a feeling of wellbeing – because you're caring for another being. That's the whole point of Connection.)

- Do something else of your choice that connects you with another human being, in person, to whom you give your undivided one-on-one attention for twenty straight minutes.

"BETTER" – PHASE TWO

Connect with a tribe and make a contribution to that tribe.

In this second phase, which builds on the first, you commit to spending at least half an hour on a group activity, during which you make some kind of personal contribution that benefits – or at least engages – the group. This goal can be big or little, silly or serious, ongoing or one-off. Pick one item from the following, list, tell your accountability partner about it – and follow through.

- Go to the gym as part of a group. Set personal and individual performance targets and compare notes when you're done. Encourage and be encouraged to take part in physical activity. Get up and out!

- Attend a religious service of your choice.

- Attend a book club.

- Attend a support group.

- With two or more people, attend a sporting event.

- With two or more people, be *part* of a sporting event. (For instance, a pickup basketball game.)

- With two or more people, visit a place you've never been before.

- Throw a party for someone at work who is underappreciated.

- Offer to babysit for someone who has two or more children.

- Do something else that gets you engaged with two or more people in real time, in person. (Going to the movies doesn't count. It's too passive.)

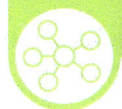

"BEST" – PHASE THREE

Take part in a charitable social activity your tribe commits to as a group.

In this third phase, which builds on the first two, you commit to spending at least an hour or two each month on a group activity where your group gives something back to the larger community. In other words, someone else who is not part of the group must directly benefit from what you and your tribe members do. So, sign up. Get involved. Give back! Pick *one* item from the following, list, tell your accountability partner about it – and follow through.

- With two or more friends, volunteer at a homeless shelter.

- With two or more friends, spend time at a nursing home, interacting with the seniors.

- With two or more friends, spend time at a hospital, interacting with the patients.

- Organize a walk-a-thon that involves two or more people you work with, and that benefits a charity you all support.

- With two or more friends, start a fund-raiser for a worthy cause. Meet in person to discuss the project.

- With two or more friends, organize a neighborhood cleanup event.

- With at least two other people, volunteer to help out at a school event.

- Working with at least two other people, get parental permission to take a local kid (or kids) out on a field trip.

- Take part in another event that involves at least two other people and benefits the larger community.

A FINAL THOUGHT ABOUT CONNECTION

This **LIVE-IT! 180°** principle is all about adding purpose to your own life and the lives of others. My request is that you never imagine that you're done with this or that you're already doing it to the degree that it needs to be done. This is literally a never-ending quest. My request is that you constantly expand your efforts to connect, to interact, and to give back. Even if you reach a point where you've got a deep sense of purpose, a point where you're doing everything I've suggested in the GOOD, BETTER, and BEST categories outlined above, you should find a way to expand the contributions you make, in person, to the lives of the people you care about, to your tribe, and to the larger human family. Find a way to give even more and connect even more.

I have had personal experience, with people I loved dearly, that convinced me that when people get complacent about connection, when they check out, when they decide it's okay to spend ten or twelve hours a day watching TV and checking Facebook, when they opt out of the world of one-on-one, in-person connection, *it's not just dangerous, it's fatal*. I've seen people I love die from this kind of lifestyle choice. It's a downhill spiral, and I've watched people I love slide down it with my own eyes. And I'm terrified when I stop to think that it's the direction our culture as a whole is headed: passive, disengaged, and waiting for electronic virtual contact instead of actual human contact.

You're never done with the job of connecting, and neither am I. The entire human family is richer for our effort to make deeper, richer, better connections with others. And we all have an obligation to look after that family.

"Come together."

—The Beatles

Plan your life and live your plan. LIVE-IT! 180°.

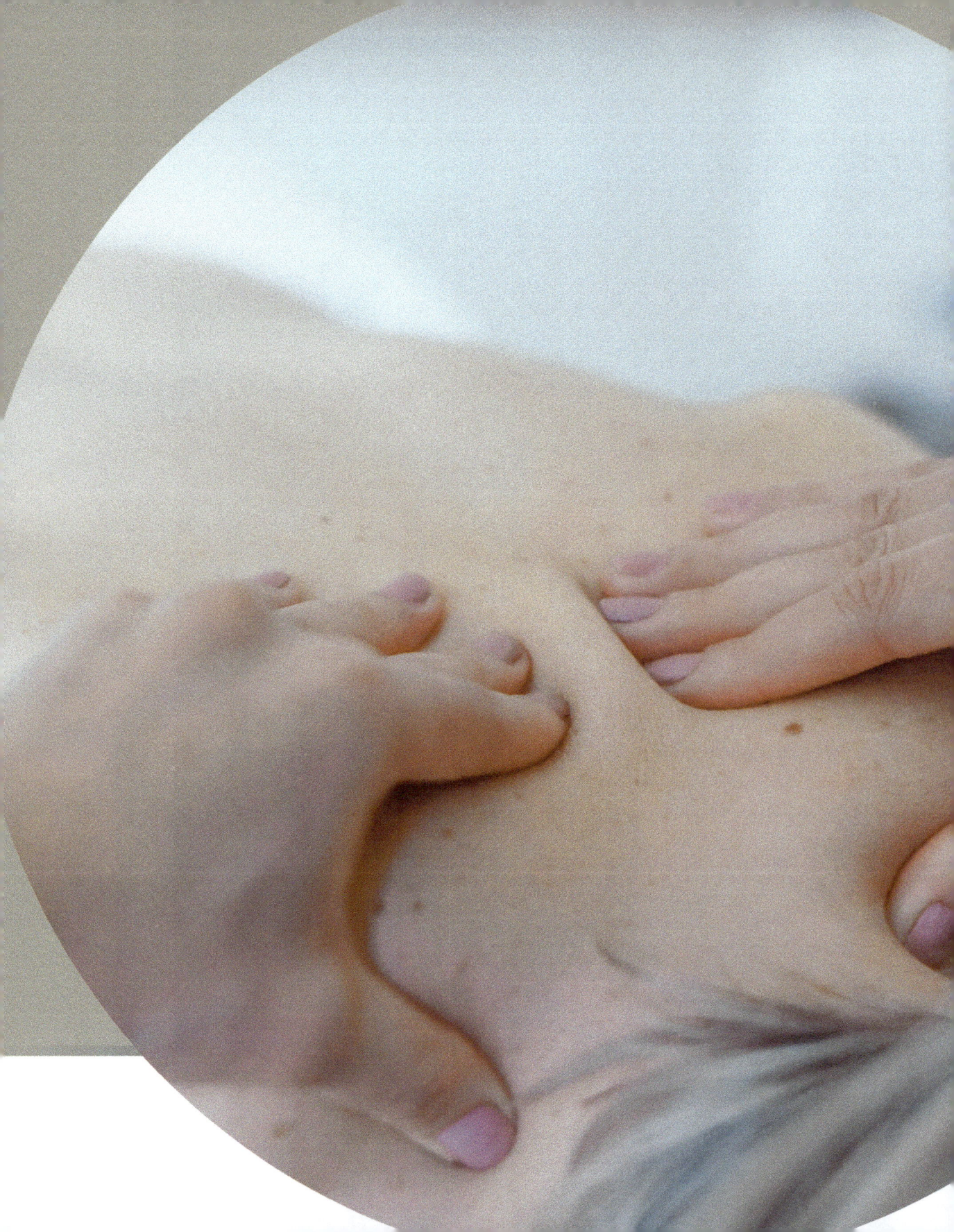

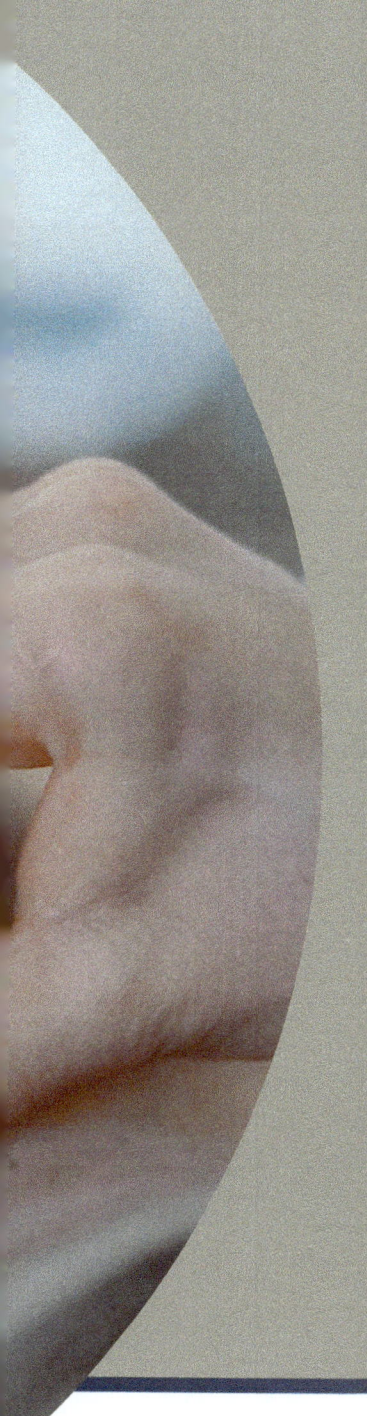

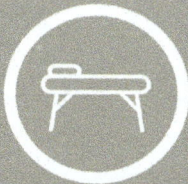

REPAIR

Remove the adverse effects of stress and wear and tear on your body by managing it effectively.

9

Remove the effects life has on your body (by managing stress effectively)

The REPAIR principle is all about getting yourself back into the natural state of balance that your Intelligent Design intended for you. It's about routine maintenance.

Recall that at the beginning of earlier chapters, I have shared with you an analogy that connected what we were working on to the "automobile" – the Intelligently Designed machine that is your astonishing human body. We've reached, in this chapter, the fifth and final piece of the puzzle – and as you surely know by now, simply understanding the five principles is only the beginning of this program. The principles are all interrelated and should all unfold in a coordinated way. (You'll see how in Chapter Ten.) The concept of interconnectedness is essential to any meaningful attempt to implement the REPAIR principle ... and it's at the heart of the last "automobile analogy" I want to share with you.

Let's assume that you're fortunate enough to own a cutting-edge high-performance vehicle that is absolutely top-of-the-line ... and brand new. Just because it's easier for us to get a sense of how serious an investment this is when we have a dollar-sign attached to the vehicle, let's say you've decided to purchase the most expensive production vehicle in the world: the Koenigsegg CCXR Trevita.

For the record, that's a $4.8 million purchase, more expensive than a top-of-the-line Lamborghini, Ferrari, or Aston-Martin. The Trevita boasts a 1000-plus horsepower V8 engine, it has a top speed of 254 miles per hour, and its body is composed of a special carbon fiber that "shines like millions of diamonds when the sun hits the car."

So, here's my question. You paid nearly five million dollars for this vehicle. Are you just going to take it out and drive it until the wheels fall off?

Would you even *consider* pushing that vehicle to its limit day after day, week after week, month after month, until something goes wrong – and only *then* taking it to a mechanic? Or would you set up a scheduled program of regular maintenance to head off problems before they arise?

> "Your health is your most valuable asset. Invest your time into taking care of it."

I hope you chose the latter option. It's obvious, isn't it? With a possession that important, representing a purchase that significant, *of course* you would schedule regular maintenance and take care of the car preventatively. That way, you would stand a better chance of *keeping* (expensive) problems from taking that valuable ride of yours off the road. With a vehicle like that, you'd be a fool *not* to keep the works tuned and lubricated at all times, *not* to check the tire pressure regularly, *not* to wash all the nooks and crannies carefully to make sure you eliminated every possible trace of salt, dirt, or grit that could damage your vehicle or adversely affect its performance. In short, instead of driving that high-performance vehicle until the wheels fell off, you'd want take account of all the effects of daily travel and deal with them before they became major issues.

That's REPAIR in a nutshell. It's a commitment you make to keep the extraordinary machine your Intelligent Design made for you in factory-showroom condition, or as close as possible to that, through a few very simple preventive-maintenance steps. I realize doing this may not be second nature to you right now, but once you make your way through the guidance you'll receive in this chapter, I think you'll find that REPAIR *becomes* second nature easily and quickly for you. Why? Because it increases your ability to perform, just like the right maintenance routine increases the ability of a world-class sports car to perform.

Understand this, though: Your body is worth *far more* than the price of a sports car – any sports car! Each of us should be *more* committed to keeping everything in our system in balance, in tune, and well cared for than we would be to keeping our car's maintenance schedule up to date. Your health is your most valuable asset. Invest your time into taking care of it.

There is a tidal wave of research out there demonstrating the debilitating effect of negative stress on the body. There is chilling evidence of the damage caused by negative stress to our systems, from simple edginess and headaches to cancer, heart disease, heart attacks, and death. Here's what you need to understand: No matter how well you sleep, no matter how sensible your food intake is, no matter how great your exercise regimen is, no matter how good your social life is, all of those things are for naught if you experience too much negative stress and don't deal constructively with it. Most people don't. And they die too early. They think dealing effectively with stress is a nice-to-have. Actually, it's a must-have. Ignoring this fundamental reality is like driving that top-of-the-line, world-class sports car without engine oil. What could go wrong? Plenty.

Maybe you think I'm exaggerating. I'm not! The best scientific research now shows us that when we allow negative stress to take the body out of balance, it upsets the natural homeostasis of the body and moves the body into a dangerous, acidic state that is basically your primal self-preservation mode. It's your fight-or-flight response. Now, this response has its place, but it's important to understand that, when your body is in this mode, it's

basically in emergency lockdown phase. It's now how you were designed to operate consistently. Yet, it's where most of us *do* operate, day after day after day. We think it's normal. It's not.

HARMFUL FOR THE ORGANISM

"Stressors comprise a long list of potentially adverse forces, which can be physical, structural, or emotional. Both the magnitude and chronicity of stressors are important... Homeostatic mechanisms, including the stress system, exert their effects in an inverted U-shaped dose – response curve (Figure 1). Basal, healthy homeostasis (or eustasis) is achieved in the central, optimal range of the curve. Suboptimal effects may occur on either side of the curve and can lead to insufficient adaptation, a state that has been called allostasis (different homeostasis) or, more correctly, cacostasis (defective homeostasis, dyshomeostasis, distress), which might be harmful for the organism in the short term and/or long term." – Source: Medscape

https://www.medscape.com/viewarticle/704866_2

When your body's divine balance is consistently overwhelmed by negative stress, it leads to a condition known as homeostatic imbalance, which is strongly correlated with diseases like diabetes, dehydration, hypoglycemia, hyperglycemia, gout, heart failure, and a wide range of conditions caused by the presence of toxins in the bloodstream. Again: Think of yourself driving that Koenigsegg CCXR Trevita down the highway at top speed, hearing the gears grind themselves down, and thinking, "I'm sure it will be fine." That's what happens when we build negative stress into our lives – degrading our own physical, mental, and structural well-being – and don't do anything to get ourselves back into a state of balance. We damage the machinery – and we reduce its useful lifespan.

EUSTRESS AND DISTRESS, REVISITED

As I've mentioned elsewhere in this book, the effects of imbalance cause what's known as *distress* on many of the body's systems. On the muscular system, for instance, negative stress can cause our muscles to tighten, knot, and develop scar tissue, adhesions, and congestion. Recall what I shared with you about this in the DRIVE chapter: When our muscles tighten or knot, they shorten. This is a problem, because muscles not only provide movement and support to the human body, they hold our vertebrae and bones together. This, in turn, protects our nerves and organs. So, guess what? Muscles that have become too short due to negative stress will move bones and vertebrae out of alignment, causing *more* stress on the nerves and a whole host of other conditions. Many of the numerous general aches and pains that everyone assumes are the effects of getting older, are actually the effects of cumulative *distress* that hasn't been dealt with – in other words, the effects of the body being out of balance.

Through muscle pliability – the act of breaking down scar tissue, adhesions, and knots – we can flush out congestion and toxins and flush in nutrients. We release the stress on the nervous system, give vital tissue and cells a healthier environment. This has huge benefits for our hormonal system. By releasing this physical stress, we release hormones that relax us and strengthen our immune system. This is just one example of how the REPAIR principle extends well beyond the area of meditation, which is only one entry point. Relaxation at each of the body's *system* levels is essential to our BIOSYMMETRY – and pliability is part of that.

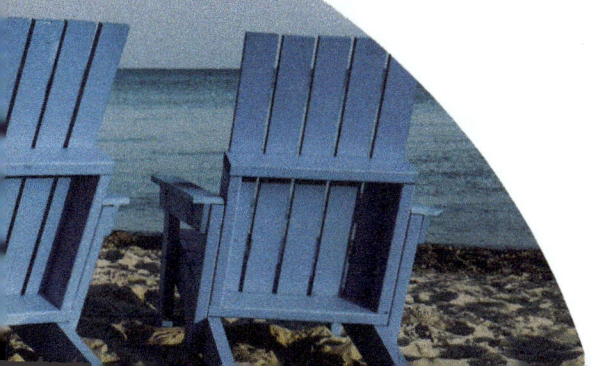

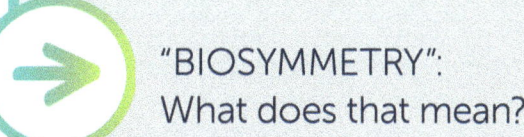

"BIOSYMMETRY": What does that mean?

Biosymmetry is a word that describes the body's natural state of balance. Getting the body back to this state of balance – through meditation, massage, and other techniques – enables all your systems to function optimally. When your system gets out of balance, there are problems. Balance in the system is restored by removing or counteracting the effects of negative stress that has accumulated at some physical, mental, or structural level.

I've shared some important information about muscle pliability and the intensive muscle and joint work necessary to bring it about because the benefits are so extraordinary, so far-reaching, and (comparatively speaking) so rapid that I've found they can have a truly remarkable impact on the overall quality of your life in the short-term, regardless of your age or your physical condition. So, this is definitely something you want to be aware of and something you want to get onto your radar screen. However, the REPAIR principle covers much more than this intensive body work, and a lot of it is far simpler and less expensive to implement.

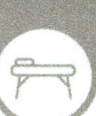

STARTING SIMPLE

As you'll see when we get to the GOOD/BETTER/BEST breakdown in this chapter, much of what you need to do in this phase of **LIVE-IT! 180°** is *ridiculously* simple. I'm predicting that you're going to read the activity items that come at the end of this chapter, and in the majority of cases, you're probably going to think to yourself, "Wow, is that all I have to do?"

And the answer, fortunately, is YES. As long as you are willing to work your way up, as long as you are willing to grow and develop and improve over time, some basic steps are all you have to take to begin the process of relaxing your body and mind. You don't have to start at the Tom Brady level, and for most people, that's as it should be. Most of us need to start very, very simple when it comes to REPAIR and then work our way up. There are two big reasons for that.

The first reason is that there are, when it comes to relaxation and stress relief, many unhelpful preconceptions for us to overcome. These preconceptions may sound like this:

- "In order to truly relax and feel balanced and comfortable in your own skin, you have to be able to meditate … and in order to be able to able to meditate, you have to be able to sit with your legs all folded up like a pretzel and recite some foreign-sounding mantra."

> "Some basic steps are all you need to take to begin the process of relaxing your body and mind."

OR:

- "In order to truly relax and feel balanced and comfortable in your own skin, you have to be able to achieve some magical, mystical, elevated state of mind or do something that's Highly Spiritual."

OR:

- "In order to truly relax and feel balanced and comfortable in your own skin, you have to be in therapy for X number of years, so you can get past whatever strange past history you have with your parents, grandparents, great-grandparents, long-lost cousins, or whoever else in your family tree you might possibly have a problem with."

Those are the typical preconceptions. I am here to tell you that not one of them is accurate. The to-do items I will share with you in this chapter are all simple enough for anyone to execute, and they don't have anything to do with meditation, Eastern mysticism, positive visualizations, or long sessions with a therapist. You can bring your body and mind into balance using the simple techniques I will be sharing with you regardless of your past history – or your lack of past history – in any of these areas. I mention this because sometimes when I tell people that REPAIR is all about getting your body and mind balanced and centered, they say things like, "You know what? I've already tried meditation, and I've found it doesn't work for me." Or, "I've spent a lot of time in therapy, and I've got relaxation down." Guess what? What I'm going to share with you here isn't meditation, it will work for you, and you can and should do it to bring yourself into balance, regardless of what has happened in your life up to this point. Literally *everyone* needs to do this and get better at it over time. But not everyone realizes that.

The second reason I've made the REPAIR principle so incredibly easy to access is this: We tend to think we're good at it, when we're really, really, really not.

I've talked about **LIVE-IT! 180°** with thousands of people over the years, and I've noticed a very interesting thing happening whenever I outline the system to someone who hasn't encountered it before. They tend to say things like, "Sleep. Got it. That's important. Eating. Got it. That's important. Drive. Got it. That's important. Connection. Got it. That's important. Repairing. That's basically chilling out, relaxing – hmm, I'm pretty sure I've got that covered." And they smile.

They really do think they have this part down already! As a result, what we typically find is that, of the five distinct, interconnected principles, REPAIR is the one that people are MOST likely to take literally no action on. Why is that? Simple. We make the mistake of believing that this principle is the same thing as whatever it is we're already doing at the end of the day to "decompress."

The challenge is, most of what we do now to "decompress" only adds to our *distress*, not to our *eustress*, in our body and mind. Most of you that do this, think that relaxation takes us *OUT* of balance. I'm talking about things like watching TV, checking our phones, eating junk food, and generally hooking up to the mass data drip that is popular culture in the twenty-first century. The corollary of all this is, in launching **LIVE-IT! 180°**, people are highly likely to make sustainable life changes in the other four areas ... and highly *unlikely* to make sustainable life changes in this one. That's a huge problem, because, as we've seen, the five principles *rely* on each other to deliver positive results to you.

REPAIR

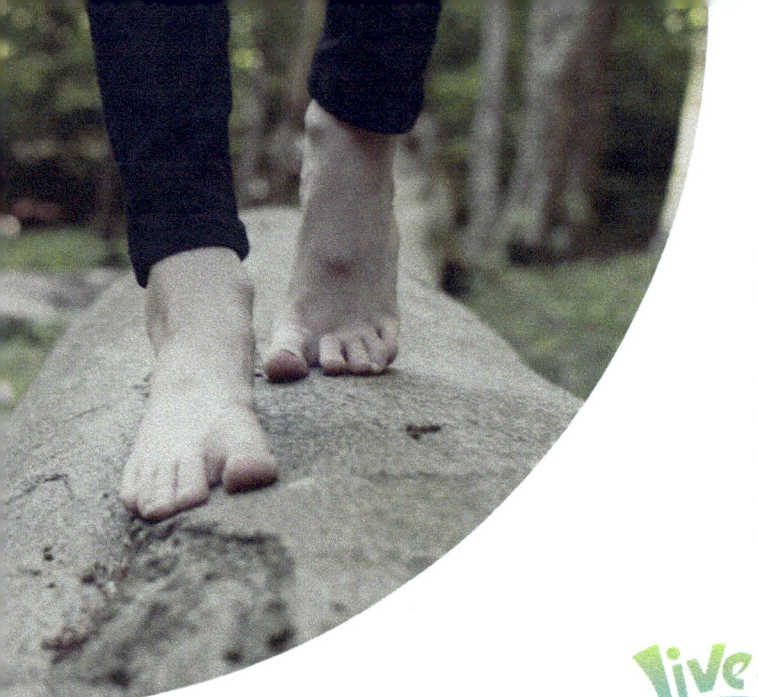

The bottom line is this: The type of "relaxing" we *think* we're really good at isn't part of the REPAIR principle. If you want to live by **LIVE-IT! 180°**, you need to do ALL of it, and that includes working your way up the GOOD/BETTER/BEST ladder you're about to read. Without that learning curve, your body and your mind are not going to be in balance, and *nothing else you do in the other four principles is going to deliver the results you deserve.*

LIVE-IT! 180° INSIGHT

Sometimes people hear about REPAIR and think to themselves – "Oh, you mean I should learn how to relax. I do that all right by myself. I'm all set with REPAIR." And they skip what follows in this chapter. Please don't be one of those people. Remember that each one of the **LIVE-IT! 180°** principles depends on your full embrace of the other four. And there's more to REPAIR than kicking back.

If just sitting back and watching TV were enough to put your system in balance, I wouldn't have needed to include a fifth **LIVE-IT! 180°** principle. But the reality is, it's not enough. And our society is worse for it. Too many of us live in a state of more or less constant negative stress. We do nothing to bring ourselves back into balance.

The GOOD/BETTER/BEST tactics you're going to read about for REPAIR all build on each other – which means you can and should keep doing the GOOD stuff as you work your way up to the BETTER and BEST stuff. In addition, they're all absolutely essential to build into your daily and weekly routine if you expect to get any lasting benefit from **LIVE-IT! 180°**.

GOOD, BETTER, **BEST**: PERSONALIZE LIVE-IT! 180°

Here's how I want you to plan your life and live your plan when it comes to the REPAIR principle. Remember, each of these levels of activity are meant to work together. Once you complete the GOOD phase and move up to the BETTER phase, you don't have to give up what's been working for you at the GOOD level. You need to build on what you've done and add to it.

"GOOD" – PHASE ONE

The first, simplest, and least expensive thing you should do to bring your body and mind into balance is called GROUNDING. What does that mean? It means every single day, you need to take five minutes, get your socks off and shoes off, and take a walk on Mother Earth. No concrete. No cement. No blacktop. Walk on the grass or the dirt, the sand, the bark mulch – anything natural and nearby and safe. Try this before you dismiss it. There is an amazing effect when your feet are bare and you're walking on dirt or grass – it really does ground you. It has a calming effect on the heart and the mind. It's as though you allow the earth to penetrate your soul for a few minutes – just by walking on it.

Cost: zero dollars. Time investment: five minutes a day. Both eminently manageable. No excuses here. Get out and do this!

The second thing I'm going to ask you to do in the GOOD category is just as simple and just as inexpensive. I want you to plan to get your more thought provoking, strenuous activities, your more stressful commitments for home and work, completed earlier in the day. Take a look at your schedule and try to plan those more challenging events so that they are all done by about two o'clock in the afternoon. Schedule the more creative and relaxed stuff for later in the afternoon. The body is better at taking care of more stressful activities in the morning because hormones like cortisol and adrenaline are firing when you first wake up. As you make your way through the day, those hormones taper off. The adrenaline goes away and more of the other sedative-like hormones kick in to get you more relaxed. Follow your body's natural rhythm and you will exert less negative stress on your body – and make it easier for you to sustain homeostasis and increase the positive stress, eustress, in the activities you do undertake.

Simple? Yes. Expensive? No. Effective? Yes. Again, no excuses. Just do this.

The third GOOD item is even simpler than the first two. Once a day, I want you to spend five minutes

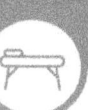

on a breather. No phones. No computers. No company. Nothing. Just take five uninterrupted minutes on your own, breathing slowly, in through your nose, out through your mouth. You don't have to recite anything (unless you want to), and you don't have to try not to think of anything. Think of whatever you want. Just breathe deeply for five minutes.

Once again: a minimal time investment, and a zero-dollar investment. There's absolutely no reason not to do this once a day, and once you get into the habit, you'll find yourself looking forward to it.

The fourth thing is equally straightforward. I want you to start each day with a written to-do list, and every time you accomplish something on it, find a simple way to celebrate. The celebration doesn't have to be fancy or expensive. It could be something as simple as listening to a favorite song. It's up to you.

Do those four very simple things every day, for at least a week, and you'll be ready to move up to the next level.

"BETTER" PHASE TWO:

Under the BETTER approach, I want you to add in something I call a 15-minute body scan. What is that? Well, I tend to do it lying in bed. Sometimes I've done it lying in the backyard or on the beach. I relax every single element of my body. I do that by taking some deep breaths, usually three to five deep breaths, then I tighten up my toes as tight as I can while I breath in deep and release them while I breath out. I then move up my body, repeating the process with my lower legs, my upper thighs, my buttocks, my stomach area, my chest, my hands, my arms, my neck, my face — taking a series of deep breaths every time. It takes about 15 minutes of deep breathing to cover everything. I finish off with three to five more deep breaths. Along the way, I notice any twinges or pains my body is trying to tell me about, and I pay attention to those. Once I get done, I'm totally relaxed. You can do this, too. How often you do this is up to you, but I'd recommend at least twice a week.

The second BETTER activity: Do a body scrub twice a week. My preferred method is to take a shower and scrub myself down with a loofa, a good sugar scrub, or a sea salt scrub, and then take a nice hot, relaxing bath. This helps to cleanse the biggest organ of our body, which is our skin.

I call the third BETTER activity "Devotions." This simply means getting outside of work, outside of family, and spending between fifteen and thirty minutes each day getting closer to your Creator.

How you do that is entirely up to you. I like reading scripture and praying. You might choose to draw or read for half an hour. It's your call. The only rule here is: No screen time during Devotions.

The fourth activity for BETTER is a once-a-week social outing of some kind. (Yes, this overlaps with CONNECT, and that's intentional.) This could be a date night with your loved one. It could be game night with your family. It could be poker night with your buddies. Whatever you choose to do, do it with two or more live human beings in real time – and make it fun for everyone. Social time is an incredibly important way to raise eustress levels and reduce negative stress (distress) levels.

After a week of making all those activities part of your routine, you're ready to expand your REPAIR repertoire by moving into …

"BEST" – PHASE THREE

(Remember, your goal here is to add to the activities you built into your schedule in the GOOD and BETTER sections.)

The number one activity at the BEST level is to get one-hour of massage and body work in from a qualified professional – ideally, someone skilled in muscle pliability work. The best schedule is once a week, but if your budget is pointing you toward once every two weeks or once a month, do that. Don't cheat yourself out of this. It is a major weapon in the war against distress. There are tons of benefits to massage, from relaxation to stress management, from releasing toxins to increasing the stimulation of your body's ability to process nutrients, from breaking down adhesions to taking care of the plaque that builds up on the muscles and the bones.

The next activity under BEST is to take care of your hands and feet. Get a manicure and/or a pedicure once a month. People who have invested the time, effort, and energy to do this know it has a massive positive effect on your quality of life and is incredibly relaxing.

The third activity at the BEST level is to increase the once-a-week social outing you got used to at the BETTER level to twice a week.

That's it!

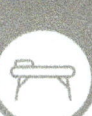

WHAT'S NEXT?

Congratulations! You now have all the core information on the five **LIVE-IT! 180°** principles. The question is, what do you *do* with that information?

I've done a lot of research on this, with the aim of identifying the very best way for you to put what you know into action, so you can make positive, long-lasting changes in your life. That research has pointed me toward a special, customizable plan for getting started with **LIVE-IT! 180°**. You'll find out all about it in the next chapter.

> *"In times of stress, the best thing we can do for each other is to listen with our ears and our hearts and to be assured that our questions are just as important as our answers."*
> —Fred Rogers

Plan your life and live your plan. LIVE-IT! 180°!

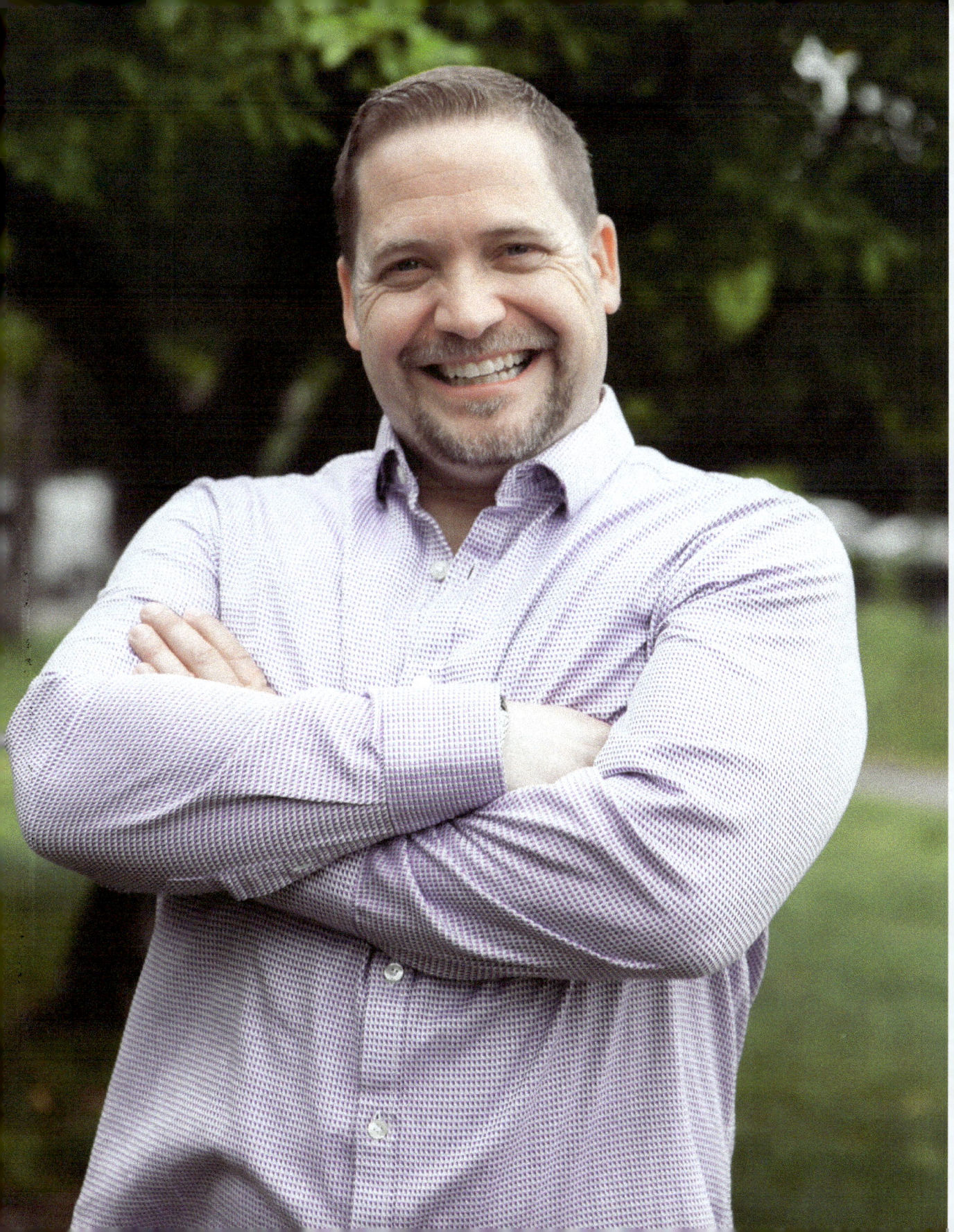

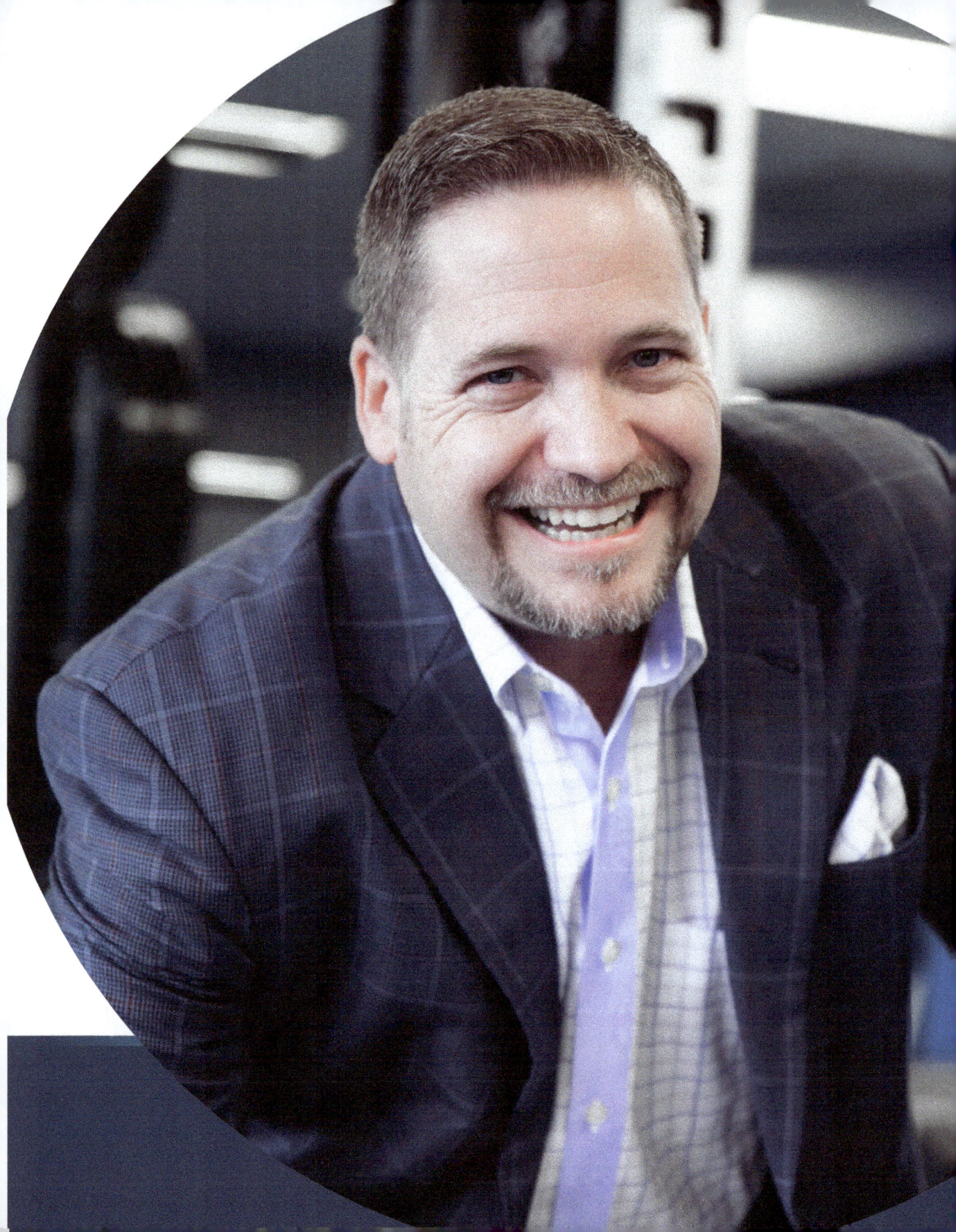

GETTING STARTED WITH THE LIVE-IT! 180° SYSTEM

10

Remaining youthful, staying fit, maintaining an ideal weight, and enjoying life – isn't this what people have wanted from life since the dawn of time? Unfortunately, we all age. That's a part of the human condition. Not only that, we are all at risk of falling into habits that accelerate the aging process and undermine those other goals. Chief among these habits are: poor sleep patterns, bad food choices, not getting enough exercise, not staying socially connected, and low-grade or non-existent stress management skills.

Put all those bad habits together, and guess what? We're gaining weight, and we're developing inflammation, disease, depression, tiredness, brain fog, toxicity, and despair ... and we're growing old before our time. However, there are steps we can take to slow down and delay that aging process, become fit, and feel good as good about ourselves as we were meant to. You've been reading about those principles in this book. Now it's time to answer the question: How do you put it all into practice?

The answer is the **LIVE-IT! 180° SYSTEM**, a carefully tested, comprehensive eight-week program that serves as your personal checklist for putting everything you've learned into practice – to enable you to attain your ideal weight, live fit, and enjoy your life..

This checklist is a simple, proven way to turn around the cumulative effect of the bad habits that are deeply woven into our modern lifestyle and tap into your body's Intelligent Design for losing weight, living fit, and enjoying life. The concept here is to implement one group of habits per week, for eight consecutive weeks, with zero regrets! This checklist gives you a few simple to-do items to focus on consistently each week. Each week you will be given a new set of habits that will build on the previous weeks' habits. By implementing those changes, establishing new habits and building on them as you go forward, you can turn things around and make dramatic, even radical, positive improvements. What I am about to share with you will help you to "do a 180 in life" – a complete change of direction, an about-face in your overall quality of life.

"The answer is the LIVE-IT! 180° SYSTEM"

Even if you've already implemented some parts of **LIVE-IT! 180°**, and it's likely you have, you can use this chapter to turn this program into an ongoing lifestyle that supports you over time. Here's my promise to you: If you use this part of the book to focus on the five areas we've covered together – Recharge, Fuel, Drive, Connect, and Repair – and if you do that consistently, over the next eight weeks, you will dramatically upgrade yourself in all those areas. You will form good habits that enable you to live according to **LIVE-IT! 180°** on autopilot. My challenge to you is:

1 – Commit to following one simple group of instructions per week, as outlined on the checklist

8 – ... for eight weeks ...

0 – ... and you'll have zero regrets.

There is no Fountain of Youth ... but fortunately there is **LIVE-IT! 180°**, which is about as close as you can expect to get.

WHY THIS IS DIFFERENT

The **LIVE-IT! 180°** system enables you to make a plan for losing weight, living fit, and enjoying life – and then live your plan. It does that in a way that actually sticks. As you've probably noticed, most "diet and exercise" implementation plans out there sound good, but they don't stick.

A lot of programs talk about their two-week or three-week jump-start. They give you that amount of time to adjust to the program and make it part of your routine.

But here's the problem: It takes four to six weeks to form a habit that becomes part of your daily life!

The **LIVE-IT! 180°** system takes this into account. It introduces just one group of new instructions per week and helps you lock them down and master them throughout the week. Each week, for eight weeks, you follow a new group of instructions, adding them to the existing ones you have implemented and made into habits, part of your life. By building core habits into your daily routine and then reinforcing them, week by week, building habit upon habit for eight straight weeks, you really can turn your life around and start losing weight, living fit, and enjoying life.

By the end of those eight weeks, you will have turned all these instructions into habits. You will have developed the skills you need, practiced them and embedded them all into your daily and weekly routine. You will have begun to recognize how **LIVE-IT! 180°** can change your life for the better – not as a fad, but as a way of life.

THREE GUIDELINES

Before you start implementing the to-do items you will find here, let's take a quick look at some guidelines you will need to follow if you want **LIVE-IT! 180°** to deliver optimum results for you.

Guideline number one – Maintain a positive mindset, no matter what happens

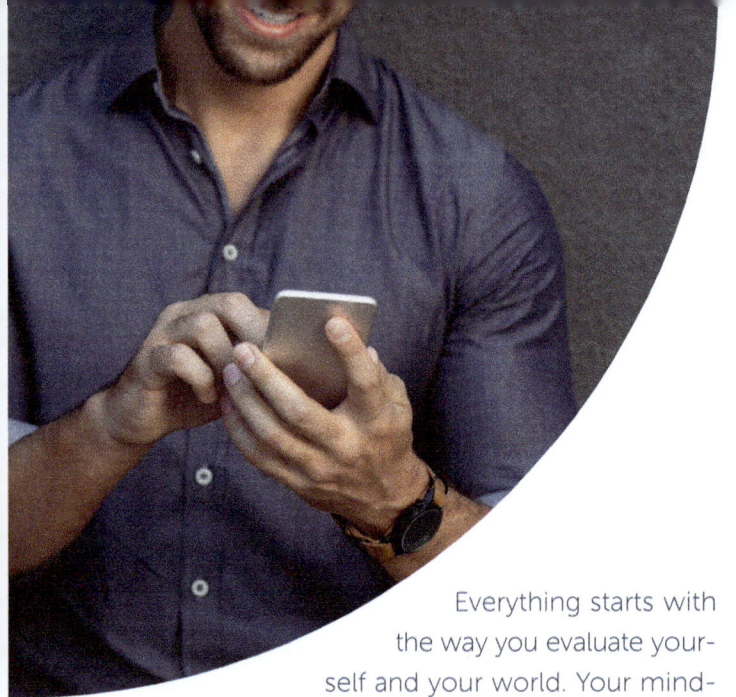

Everything starts with the way you evaluate yourself and your world. Your mindset needs to be one of "I can do this, and I will do this." This is a marathon, not a sprint, and you're going to face challenges along the way. However, if for some reason you slip and fall down along the way, your mindset should be optimistic enough to allow you to get right back up and keep moving forward. Remember, you are changing decades of bad habits. There is no quick solution. Everybody stumbles now and then. Nonetheless, maintaining positive forward momentum is still something you can and will make happen over the next eight weeks.

Guideline number two – Set time aside to plan

We set up a plan when we go to work. We set up a plan when we go to the movies with our friends. We set up a plan when we go to the doctor. We set up a plan when we have a Thanksgiving dinner. We plan all these things in enough detail to achieve whatever it is we mean to achieve …. but for some reason we never stop and plan when it comes to maximizing our greatest asset, which is our health. That has to change! So, we're going to devote a certain amount of time, one day a week, to the all-important task of planning out the week ahead and preparing for it. I'll give you more details on how to do this as we look at the individual weeks. For the moment, I just want you to get used to the idea of investing a certain amount of time each Sunday on planning ahead. Think of Sunday as your planning day.

By the way: If you find yourself resistant to this idea, let me ask you a question. Suppose I wanted to get from Boston, Massachusetts, to San Francisco, California. If I just jumped in my car and started to drive without a map, a guide, a suitcase, money, or any of the other resources I would need for the trip, how far do you think I would get? Well, if my car has a full tank when I start out, I'm only going to get about 400 miles … and then I'm done. I'm lost. I have no fuel and no idea where I am and where I should go next. I may have a basic sense of direction, but there is simply no way I'm going to get to San Francisco if I haven't taken a little time up front to create my plan of attack.

Our life is both a destination and a journey. We need to identify a destination and then plan the journey. That's what I'm going to help you to do … starting on the first Sunday that you commit yourself to following **LIVE-IT! 180°**.

Guideline number three – Formalize your arrangement with your accountability partner

It's possible you've already done this, and if you

have, that's great. If not, do it now. There needs to be someone you check in with on a daily basis to discuss how you're doing on the plan. (If you want, we can be your accountability partner. Visit us at www.liveit180.com for details.) It's better if your accountability partner is also doing the **LIVE-IT! 180° SYSTEM**, but it's not mandatory. Yet you must *have* an accountability partner.

I can't emphasize this point enough. If you want **LIVE-IT! 180°** to work, this is non-negotiable. No ifs, ands, or buts. You must have an accountability partner, whether it's us here at **LIVE-IT! 180°**, or your spouse/significant other, or your next-door neighbor, or whoever you choose. Build that relationship in and remember that your accountability partner has to understand the role he or she is playing.

With those three guidelines in mind, let's get started. It's time to change your lifestyle – and help you become the you that you were designed to be.

LIVE-IT! 180° TIP

If you don't yet have an accountability partner, reach out to us at www.liveit180.com. We help people make it through the LIVE-IT! 180° systems with a high rate of success. You'll learn about the LIVE-IT! 180° app, which will provide you with daily and weekly reminders, one-on-one coaching interactions that keep you accountable and on track, and advice on how best to overcome the obstacles you face.] The app is available at the iTunes Store and the Google Play store.

1 LIVE-IT! 180° – WEEK ONE

It's possible that you're already doing something that connects to one of the habits that I mention here. Even if that's the case, do not jump ahead to the next week. Simply execute what you're supposed to execute, week by week, just as it's laid out here. If that means you keep doing something that's already familiar to you, great. Use that week to lock that habit down even stronger than it's locked down now.

Week One, Habit One: Sunday Prep 101, Journal

Congratulations. This is the week you begin to say goodbye to Ghost Food!

You'll recall that in Chapter Six, FUEL, I told you that you would have two weeks to consume all the mainstream Big Food products that are in your pantry right now. Guess what? That two-week transition period starts THIS SUNDAY ... and it begins with a simple shopping-list planning session. You will need to give this task between thirty and sixty minutes of uninterrupted time.

Again: You don't have to throw away any of the Ghost Food that's already in your possession. You just want to begin the process of finishing it all off this week. So, make written plans, starting this Sunday, to REPLACE each unhealthy food item in your kitchen with a healthier alternative, following the guidelines laid out in Chapter Six.

Record, in a journal of your choice, the shopping list you will use to begin your two-week transition period. For instance, if you have a quart of cow's milk in the fridge, you might make a note to replace that with a quart of almond milk the next time you go shopping. Get it all down in black and white. Make a complete shopping list for this week based on the approach you chose for yourself in Chapter Six.

You should also use your Sunday Prep time to get used to the "hand portion" measurement system that you learned about in Chapter Six. If you haven't familiarized yourself with that system and with what it means for your personal weekly food intake, use your Sunday Prep time to get familiar enough with it, know what you will need for quantity, and create your first **LIVE-IT! 180°** shopping list.

Remember: Starting this Sunday, anything new that goes into your pantry needs to match up with one of these three FUEL approaches: the GOOD approach (page XX), the BETTER approach (pages XX), or the BEST approach (page XX).

What you actually eat this week is still entirely up to you. You can finish whatever Ghost Food you already own and feel like eating. Just notice what you're eating ... plan to replace it with something better whenever you can ... and remind yourself that you won't be buying processed food anymore. At the end of Week Two, any processed food that remains goes into the garbage can!

If you have already finished your two-week transition period and completed your Kitchen Makeover, you can simply move on to...

Week One, Habit Two: H20verhaul

If you haven't done so already, this is the week you will begin to follow **LIVE-IT! 180°** in terms of your personal daily water consumption. Yes, this is a higher water intake than most people are initially used to. Stay with it. Your body and comfort level will adjust. Remember not to drink water too close to bedtime, otherwise you will disrupt your sleep patterns.

This week, you will make a point of drinking "half your body's weight" in pounds every day – by translating the pounds of your body weight into ounces of water, and then dividing by two. For example, a person who weighs 180 pounds would drink 90 ounces of water each day.

Week One, Habit Three: Sleep ... the Final Frontier

This week, you will schedule your days and evenings in such a way that you guarantee yourself at least seven and a half consecutive hours of uninterrupted sleep.

Follow the guidelines in Chapter Five to make sure this happens.

WEEK ONE SUMMARY

1. Sunday Prep 101 / Journal / Shopping List

2. Daily H2O Intake (½ your body weight in ounces)

3. Sleep 7.5 to 9 hours every night

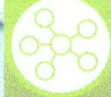

# LIVE-IT! 180° – WEEK TWO

In Week Two, you will continue to adopts the habits you locked down in Week One, and you will begin to lock down three more critical **LIVE-IT! 180°** habits. They are:

Week Two, Habit One: Sunday Prep SECOND LEVEL, Life Plan

This is the week you COMPLETE the process of saying goodbye to Ghost Food!

Give yourself between thirty and sixty minutes this Sunday to create the shopping list that replaces all the Ghost Food that you will consume this week with healthier alternatives. (This is a continuation of what you started in Week One.)

Remember that, by the end of this week, you will need to throw out any food that does not match up with the GOOD, BETTER, or BEST approach you selected at the end of Chapter Six. Be sure you have replacement groceries in stock that will allow you to make the transition to that eating plan, beginning on Sunday of next week.

In addition, you should use your Sunday Prep time to map out, briefly but clearly, all your anticipated time investments for the entire week to come. For instance, you should block off – in your journal, datebook, or calendar applications – the specific time that you will go to sleep each night, and the specific time that you will wake up each day. You should block off all your work time, all your leisure time, all your travel time, and so forth. This will become second nature, but for now please, please, please do this!

Week Two, Habit Two: Vital Veggies

Eat one to two proper hand portions of fresh and/or cooked vegetables at every meal every day this week, following the "hand" guidelines laid out in Chapter Six. Target 3 meals a day.

Examples of foods you can eat in support of this habit include broccoli, cauliflower, spinach, and Romaine lettuce. Please check the shopping list provided in the Appendix that appears at the end of this book. Mix up your veggie choices. My favorite is roasted broccoli.

Week Two, Habit Three:
Protein Power

Eat one proper hand portion of protein with every meal each day this week, following the guidelines laid out in Chapter Six. Target three meals a day.

Examples of foods you can eat in support of this habit include beans, eggs, chicken, fish, beef, and pork (as long as it is high quality pork with no nitrates/nitrites). I would caution you to not have bacon and sausage every day. Mix up your protein choices.

Remember to continue sticking to the previous week's habits. (Sunday Prep, Shopping List, H2O Daily Intake, Sleep) You can do this!

WEEK TWO SUMMARY

1. Ghost Food Out / Life Plan

2. Veggies 3 times a day
   (1-2 whole hands)

3. Protein 3 times a day
   (1 palm of hand)

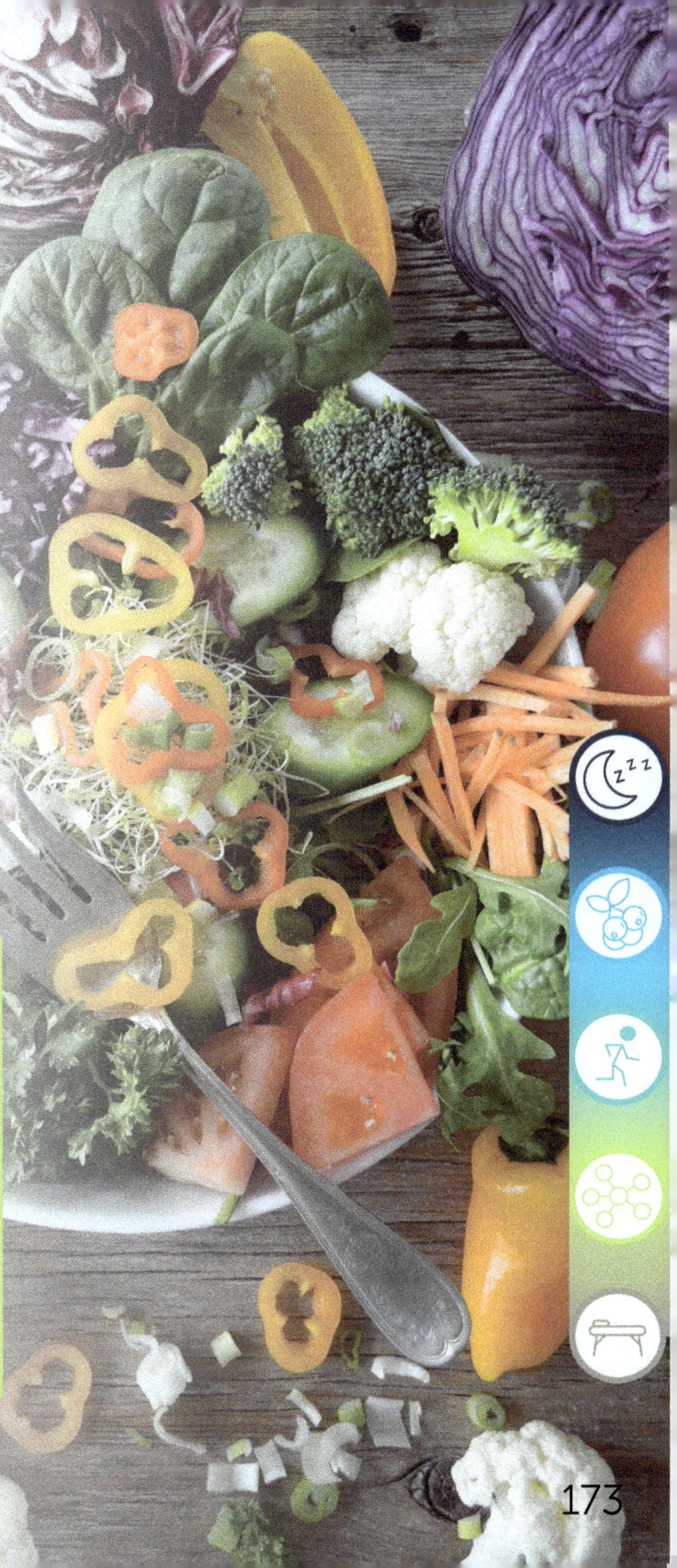

LIVE-IT! 180° – WEEK THREE

In Week Three, you will maintain all the habits you learned in Weeks One and Two, and you will begin to establish three more critical **LIVE-IT! 180°** habits.

Week Three, Habit One: Sunday Prep ADVANCED LEVEL, Meal Planning

Woo hoo! Starting today, you are operating in a kitchen that is entirely free of Ghost Food! It's very important that you complete and celebrate this benchmark. Schedule some kind of appropriate personal reward time for yourself for doing this!

Use your Sunday Prep time this week not only to create your next shopping list, but also to prepare specific foods you will consume over the next seven days. For instance, if you know you are going to eat one hard-boiled egg a day for the next seven days, use your Sunday Prep time to boil seven hard-boiled eggs. If you plan to eat five servings of chopped raw carrots over the coming week, use your Sunday Prep time to get as many of those servings ready as you can. Get into the routine of prepping as much of your food ahead of time as you can, based on how long it will last once you've prepped it. (By the way, if you do this with a spouse or partner, it definitely counts as Connect time.)

Of course, you should also use the Sunday Prep time to plan out your life plan schedule for the coming week, as you began doing in Week Two. Remember, each habit you master in **LIVE-IT! 180°** should continue to be part of your routine as you move forward.

Week Three, Habit Two: Fat – That's Good!

Not all fat is created equal. If you've made it this far in the book, you already know that you need good fat to survive. Good fat is the lubricant of the Intelligently Designed machine that is your body. So, starting this week, you're going to begin consuming one serving of good fat at each of your three meals. Do you remember how much you should eat at each sitting? That's right: Enough to equal the volume of your thumb, from the tip of your thumb down to where it meets your palm. Foods that fall into the "good fat" category include avocado, olive oil, coconut, nuts, and seeds.

Week Three, Habit Three: Movement Meal Bonus

For each thirty-minute session of appropriate vigorous movement you complete during a given day, give yourself one extra palm-sized serving of protein and one extra thumb-sized serving of good fat at the next meal. ("Vigorous movement," also known as exercise, is something you can define for yourself, in consultation with your physician. It's physical activity that elevates your heart rate and/or places resistance on your muscles, such as a muscle workout at the gym, cardio on a bike, or a fast walk up the street. My guess is you already know what this is – and isn't – in your world.)

Continue with the previous week's habits: Sunday Prep, Shopping List, Life Plan, H2O Daily Intake, Sleep, Veggies, and Protein. You can do this!

WEEK THREE SUMMARY

1. Meal Planning

2. Fats

3. Movement Meal Bonus

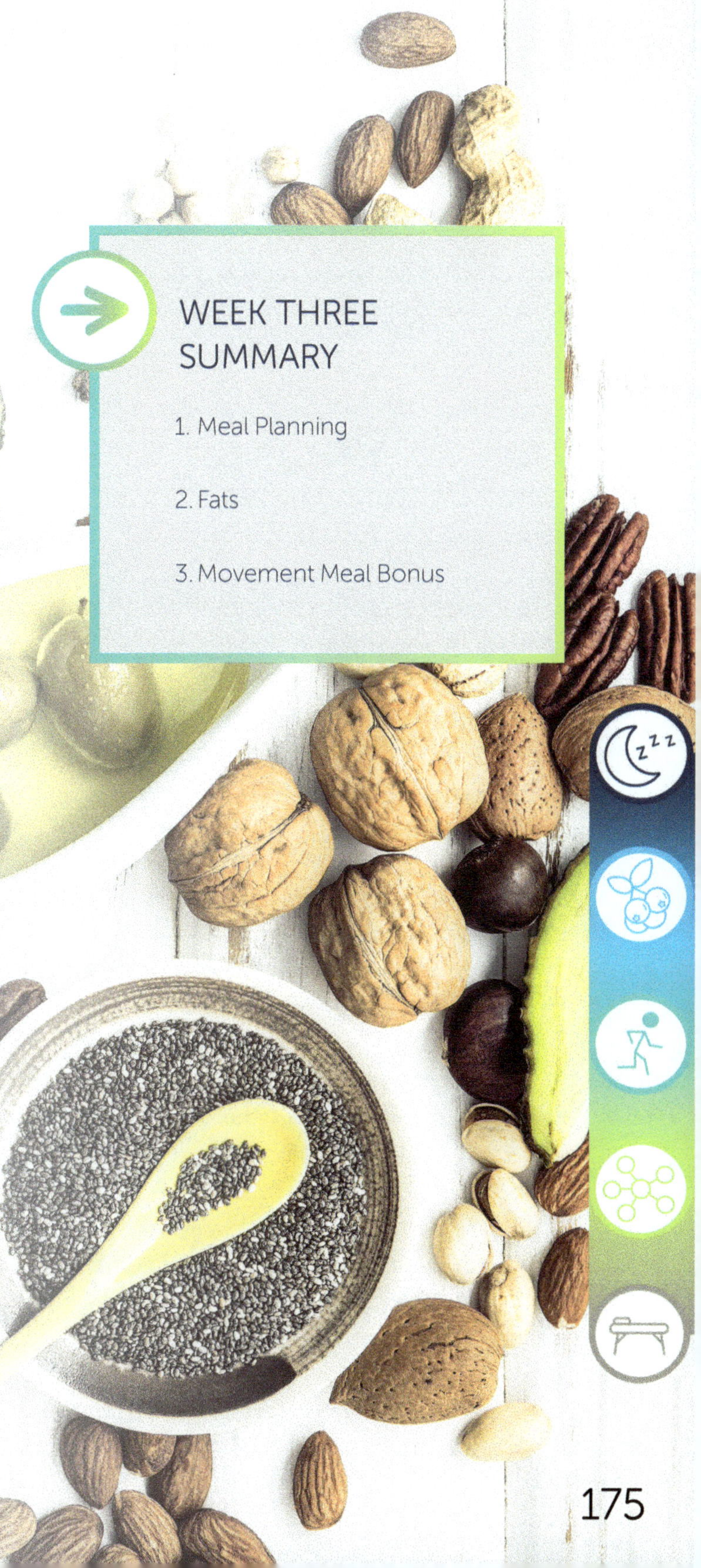

# LIVE-IT! 180° – WEEK FOUR

In Week Four, you will continue following the habits I shared with you in Weeks One, Two, and Three (including the advanced phase of your Sunday Prep - Meal Planning), and you will also adopt two more critical **LIVE-IT! 180°** habits, each of which connects to the DRIVE principle. Note: Review your personal exercise plan with your physician before you start executing either of these habits.

Week Four, Habit One: Don't Be Uptight – Do the Five-Minute Stretch

Once a day, spend five consecutive minutes doing some basic stretching moves. This can be as simple as getting a lacrosse ball and putting it under the ball of your foot while you stand and put most of your weight on that foot, working the ball back and forth slowly along the length of the foot. You're likely to find some areas that feel a little tender. Those are trigger points – push down on them with slowly graduated pressure so you can get a nice strong stretch. Do this for two and a half minutes on one foot. Then do the same thing on the other foot.

Another great option is to do your stretches with a foam roller. Sitting on the ground (or on an exercise mat), support yourself with your palms, put the roller under one leg, and roll your leg back and forth. Sitting on the roller, start by working on your calves, then on your hamstrings, then on your quads, then on your tailbone. Then work the other leg in the same way. You can add in side-rolling on your obliques as well as your neck. Check out liveit180.com for our foam rolling videos and demonstrations.

If you don't have either of those resources and don't feel like getting them, you can just stand comfortably and shake out/stretch out your legs, back, neck, and arms in a way that feels comfortable for you.

Whatever you decide to do as a daily stretching routine, do it for five consecutive minutes each day.

IMPORTANT: I've given you the barest outline of the Five-Minute Stretch. For a more detailed plan that you can personalize to your own unique situation, and for coaching on that plan, visit liveit180.com.

Week Four, Habit Two: 15/3/6

For fifteen minutes a day, three days out of every seven, do these six forms of exercise: bend, squat, push, pull, plank, and pump. Notice that you should adapt each exercise to your own capacity, in consultation with your doctor.

- BEND: One way to do this is to make sure your feet are a shoulder-width apart, then pushing your butt back and keeping your chest straight, reach down to the floor, touch it, and come right back up again. For most healthy adults, I recommend 20 repetitions, but you'll want to adapt this to what feels right for you.

- SQUAT: The same basic idea, only instead of bending your back and touching the floor with your hands, you keep your spine straight and squat down as low as you can comfortably go. Then stand back up again, keeping your stomach tight the whole time. Target 20 repetitions and increase as you progress.

- PUSH: For some people, this is a simple, standard, classic military push-up. Others prefer to do the push-up from the knees upward. Others lie against a wall at an angle and then push themselves away from the wall. Basically, it's anything that you want to do and feel comfortable doing that involves pushing your body away from a surface. Again, 20 repetitions is standard.

- PULL: There are countless variations on this one, the basic idea of which is simple: pull something towards you. One simple, customizable approach is to fill up a water jug to a level that feels right and use the jug to do bicep curls. A more aggressive take on this exercise pattern is the classic pull-up. There are lots of variations using exercise bands too. Pick something you can do 20 times – and do it!

- PLANK: A great beginner's version of this core-strengthening move is to rest your forearms and toes on a towel or mat and hold the rest of your body stiff for 20 seconds. (The advanced version does the same thing, but from the same arms-extended position you'd use at the beginning of a classic push-up. Keep your belly tucked and sides tight.)

- PUMP: This is probably the simplest exercise of the bunch. Do twenty jumping jacks, at a speed that you feel comfortable with. Get the heart pumping.

That's the new habit! Do all of six of those exercises, three times a week, for a total of fifteen minutes per session. You'll get your heart pumping, keep your joints flexible, and strengthen your core. Keep it up! You'll notice after only a few weeks that your body starts yearning for the exercise, and you'll look forward to the sessions.

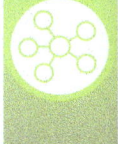
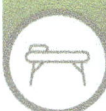

IMPORTANT: I've given you just the barest outline of the 15/3/6 exercise plan. For a much more detailed plan that you can personalize to your own unique situation, and for coaching on that plan, visit liveit180.com.

As a reminder, continuing to follow the previous week's habits. (Sunday Prep, Shopping List, Life Plan, Meal Planning, H2O Daily Intake, Sleep, Veggies, Protein, Fats, and Movement Meal Bonus) You are doing great. Keep it going!

WEEK FOUR SUMMARY

1. 5 Minute Stretch

2. 15/3/6

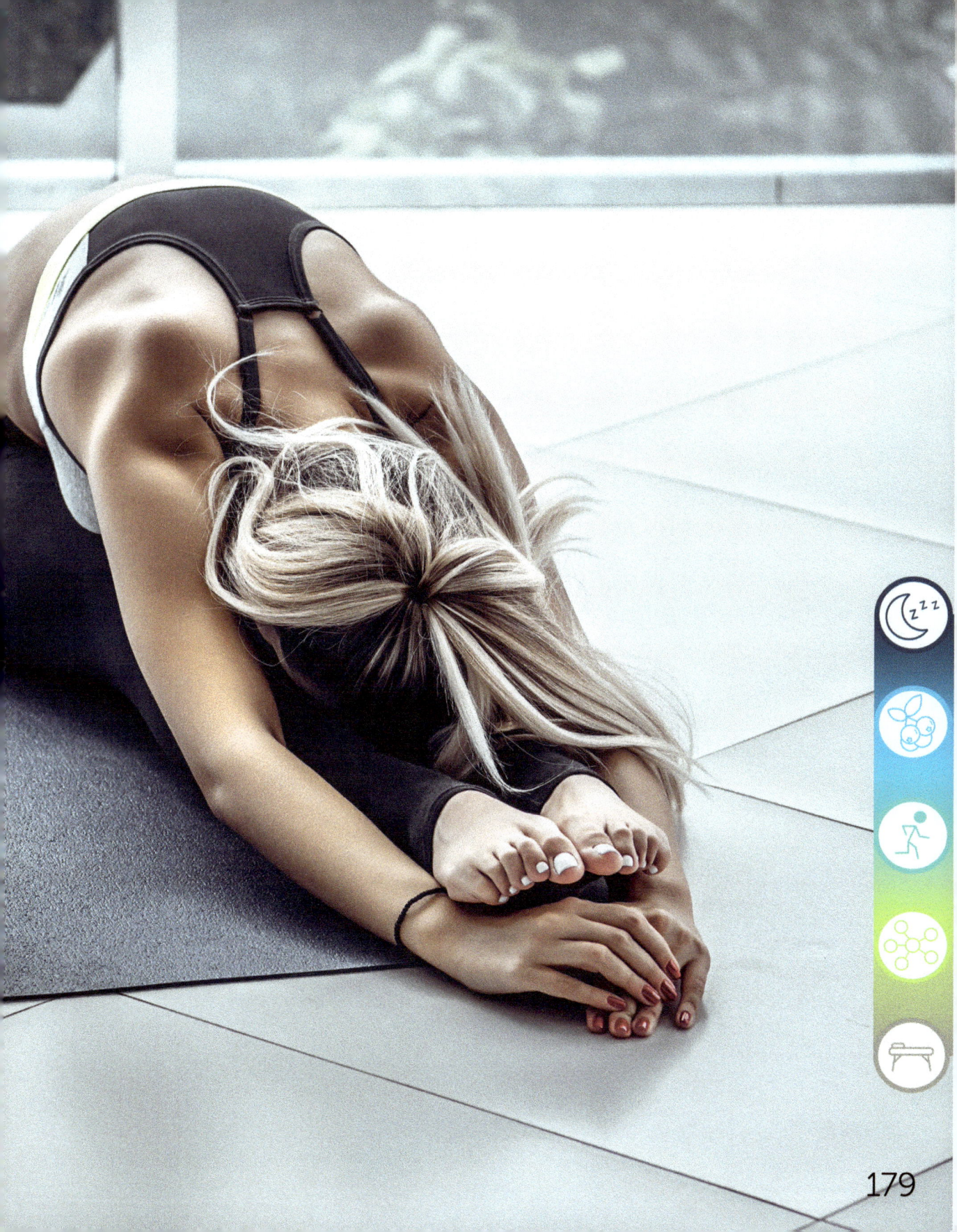

 # LIVE-IT! 180° – WEEK FIVE

In Week Five, you will keep up all the habits you learned about in Weeks One, Two, Three, and Four, and you will also begin to master two more critical **LIVE-IT! 180°** Habits. (That's right – just two new habits. The new-habit load begins to get a little lighter from this point forward for a simple reason: You're not just adopting one new week's worth of new habits, but all the habits of all the weeks that have you have learned, as well!)

Week Five, Habit One: Family/Friend Time

Each week, from today, you are going to schedule and participate in one face-to-face, non-work-related social activity involving at least one other person (if you can get two other people, that would be even better). I don't care what this social activity involves, but you must spend at least ninety minutes or more doing it. The possibilities are endless: book club, poker night, movie night, bowling night. The only rules are that it must not be about work and it must involve real human beings, in the same room with you, in real time, for at least an hour and a half.

This would include a conversation with your spouse or significant other right in the middle of your kitchen. No texting. No posting a one-way video on Facebook that other people comment on. To fulfil this habit, you have to be able to hear each other and finish each other's sentences. If you schedule a daily check-in with your accountability partner, and then follow through on that, you're good to go.

A reminder: Continue with the previous week's habits: Sunday Prep, Shopping List, Life Plan, Meal Planning, H2O Daily Intake, Sleep, Veggies, Protein, Fats, Movement Meal Bonus, 5 Min Stretch, and 15/3/6. You are doing great, keep it going!

Week Five, Habit Two: The Daily Connect

Every day, reach out to a real, live human being, whom you like, and have a conversation about any topic you both feel comfortable with for at least ten minutes. This one can be done at a distance, as long as you can hear the other person's voice.

WEEK FIVE SUMMARY

1. Family/Friend Time

2. Daily Connect

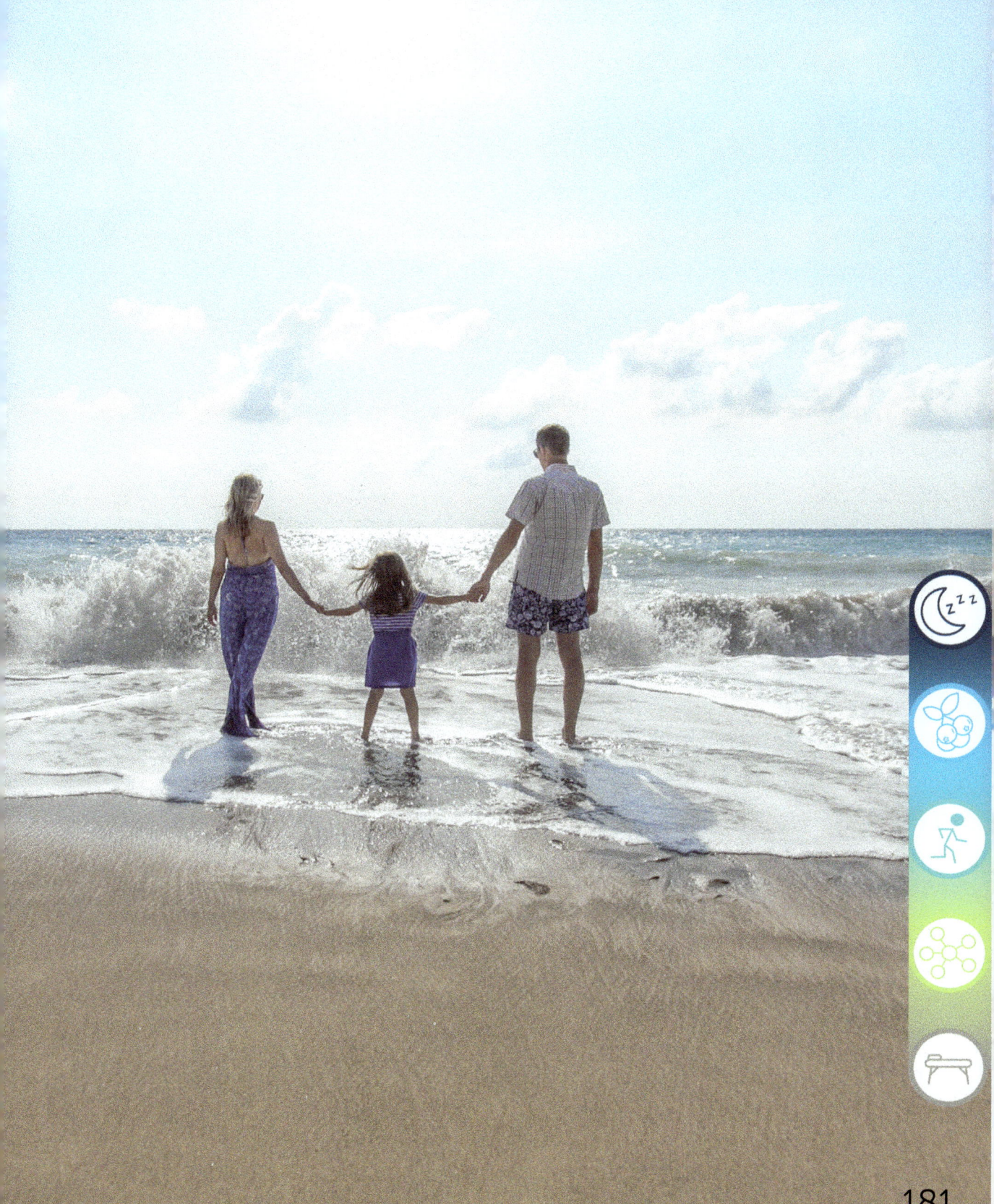

6 LIVE-IT! 180° – WEEK SIX

In Week Six, you will continue with the habits you locked down in Weeks One, Two, Three, Four, and Five, and you will also begin to implement two more critical *LIVE-IT! 180°* Habits. (Again – just two new habits. They're simple, and they require minimal time commitments, so they'll be easy to add to everything you're doing already in LIVE-IT! 180°.)

Week Six, Habit One: "Me Time"

Each week, take at least half an hour of personal time for yourself, time that does not involve interactive media in any way, shape, or form. This could be reading a book, going hiking, or taking the dogs for a walk. It can be anything that you (a) do on your own and (b) smile as you do it. Don't say you don't have time to build this habit into your schedule, because you do. If you can't find 30 minutes in the course of an average week, I'm going to go out on a limb and suggest that you may be mindlessly grazing away at Facebook, Twitter, YouTube, or similar platforms for long stretches of time.

I like to do my daily devotions during "me time." However, that's up to you. Remember, I am only asking you to schedule and spend thirty minutes a week on this habit. If you want to do something daily, great! This "Me Time" is the foundation to de-stressing and balancing your life/hormones/work so you can enjoy the benefits of reduced stress and a mind free of technology.

Week Six, Habit Two: The Three-Minute Breather

Each day, take three minutes of private time to lie down flat on your bed, relax, and take extremely deep, cleansing breaths. As you do this, notice where there is stress or discomfort in your body, and use the exhale of the next deep breath to release that stress or discomfort. This is a time to be alone and mindful of what is actually taking place in your body. Again, if you think you don't have time for this, I have a question for you: Do you have three minutes a day to follow the latest meaningless celebrity gossip and drama online? I thought so. Reassign those three minutes to this habit. You will center your mind and your spirit, and you will begin to look forward to these three precious minutes of complete calm. I tend to do this lying in bed, in the morning, just after waking up.

Remember: Continue with the previous week's habits: Sunday Prep, Shopping List, Life Plan, Meal Planning, H2O Daily Intake, Sleep, Veggies, Protein, Fats, Movement Meal Bonus, 5 Min Stretch, 15/3/6, Family/Friend Time, and Daily Connect. You are doing great, keep it going!

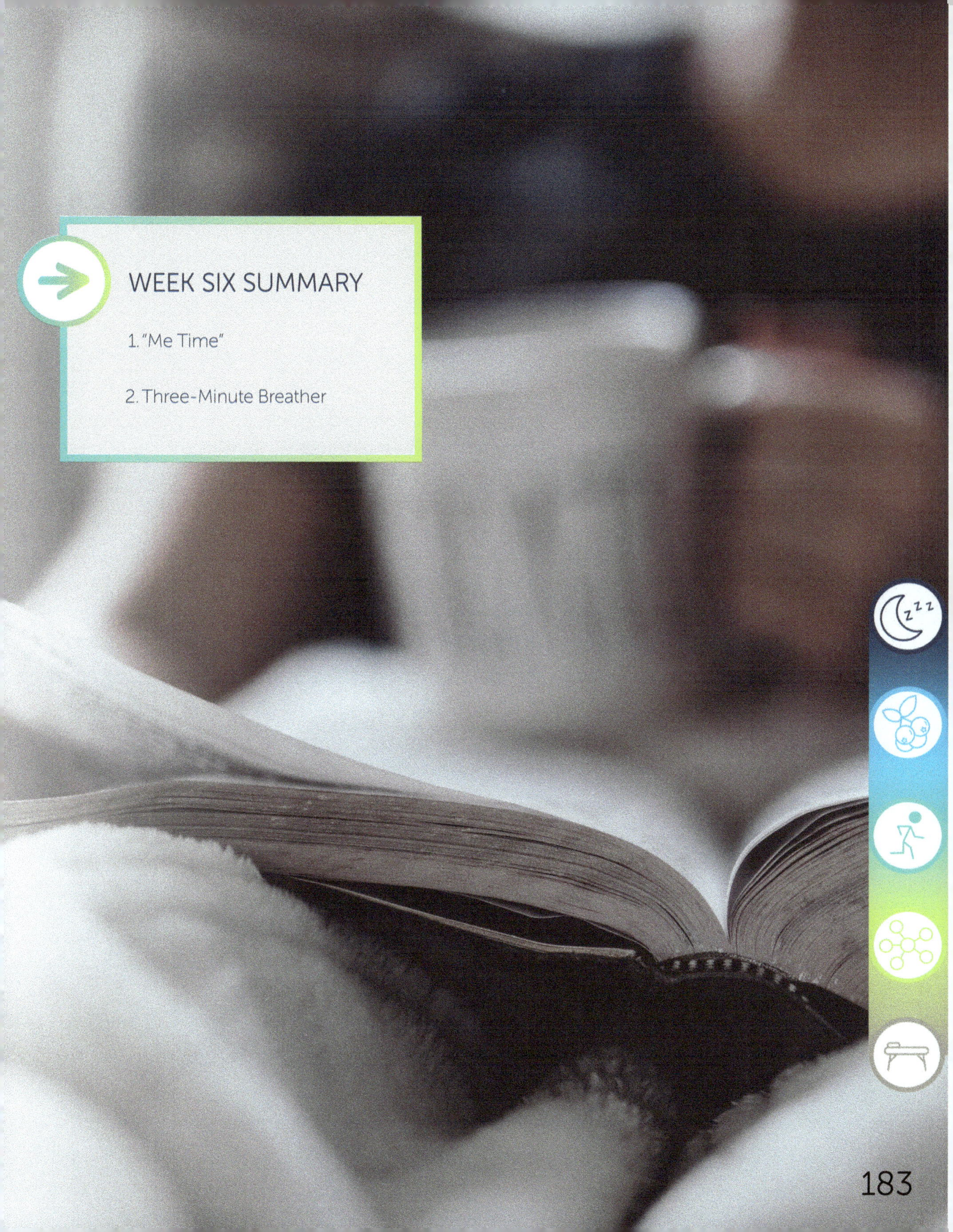

WEEK SIX SUMMARY

1. "Me Time"

2. Three-Minute Breather

LIVE-IT! 180° – WEEK SEVEN

In Week Seven, you will continue with all the habits you started in Weeks One through Six, and you will also start investing time in two more critical **LIVE-IT! 180°** Habits. The first focuses on our Intelligently Designed capacity to learn and grow, no matter how old we are. (This habit covers both the CONNECT and REPAIR principles of **LIVE-IT! 180°**.) The second habit reinvigorates your body. (It relates to the REPAIR principle of **LIVE-IT! 180°**.)

Week Seven, Habit One: Tribal Learning

Each week, I want you to spend thirty minutes in a class that involves personal interactions with others, which teaches you something you didn't know before. This could be a cooking class, a history class, a yoga class, a dance class – anything that engages you, expands your knowledge and experience base, and involves real-time interaction with other individuals.

Week Seven, Habit Two: Skin Deep

Each week, take the time to do something wonderful for your skin. Your skin is the largest, and I would add, the most commonly overlooked, organ in your body. Once a week, you're going to do something wonderful for this organ. This could involve scrubbing all those dead cells off with a salt or sugar scrub while you're in the shower. It could be a weekly massage. Or it could be something else, like a pore-cleansing masque treatment, a manicure, or a pedicure. There are plenty of possibilities. Find one that fits your budget – then treat yourself!

Do not overlook these two habits. There are the areas in which most people miss in their walk of life/health. Many put them off, or worse, don't see the need for them. Trust me, this will make one of the best, deepest, and most meaningful contributions to your overall happiness, healthiness, and feelings of youthfulness.

Reminder: Continue with the previous week's habits: Sunday Prep, Shopping List, Life Plan, Meal Planning, H2O Daily Intake, Sleep, Veggies, Protein, Fats, Movement Meal Bonus, 5 Min Stretch, 15/3/6, Family/Friend Time, Daily Connect, "Me Time", and 3 Min Breather. You are doing great, keep it going!

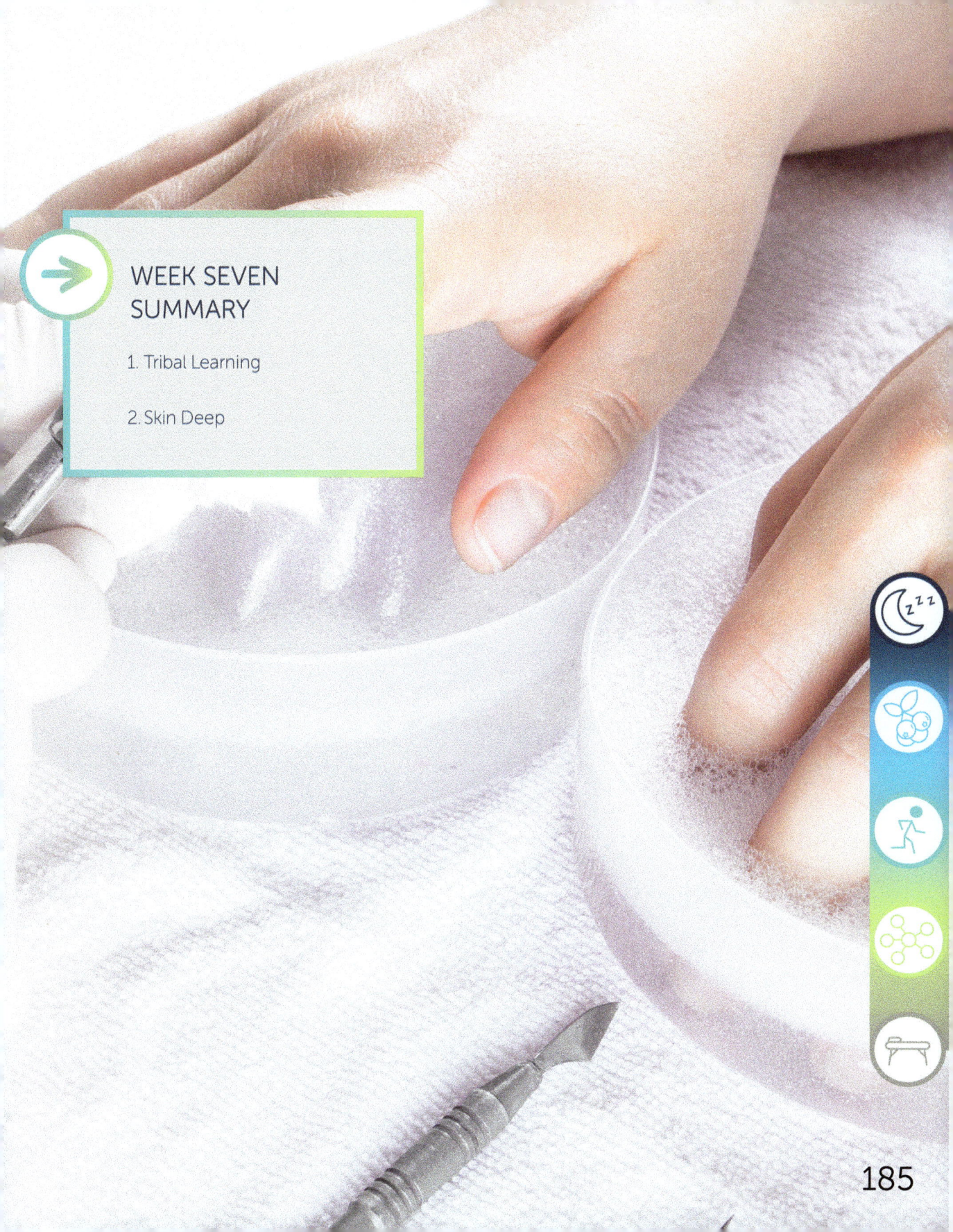

WEEK SEVEN SUMMARY

1. Tribal Learning

2. Skin Deep

LIVE-IT! 180° – WEEK EIGHT

As you wrap up your eighth week on the **LIVE-IT! 180°** system, you will keep up all the habits you started in Weeks One through Seven – and you will add one final habit to the mix as you make your victory lap. By now, if you've followed through on everything I've shared with you so far, I'm betting you will decide that some, or maybe all, of these habits belong in your life on a permanent basis. Remember, that's the idea of this system, to develop *habits* that will enable you to lose weight, live fit, and enjoy life.

Week Eight, Habit One: Supplements: An Easy Task to Swallow

Take a daily vitamin supplement that provides you with all the vitamins and minerals you need. Be sure it's made from whole food, not from synthetics. (We strongly recommend Megafood, which meets these criteria. Most supplements don't.) Take a daily probiotic supplement, made from live bacteria, to support intestinal health and immunity. (Again, we strongly recommend Megafood, which meets these criteria; most probiotics don't.) Follow the other suggestions I made in the supplement section.

IMPORTANT: Customizing your supplement intake is extremely important. The needs of a man differ from those of a woman. What you need when you're 20 is likely to be different from what you need when you're 60. For help in putting together a customized supplement plan that supports your personal health at your time of life, visit us at liveit180.com, and we'll help you get set up.

Remember: Continue with the previous week's habits: Sunday Prep, Shopping List, Life Plan, Meal Planning, H2O Daily Intake, Sleep, Veggies, Protein, Fats, Movement Meal Bonus, 5 Min Stretch, 15/3/6, Family/Friend Time, Daily Connect, "Me Time", 3 Min Breather, Tribal Learning, and Skin Deep. You are doing great, keep it going!

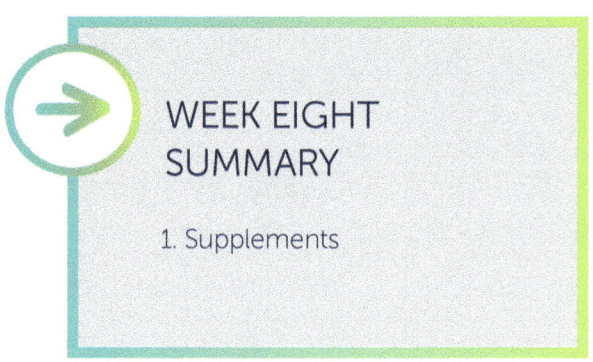

WEEK EIGHT SUMMARY

1. Supplements

That's it! That's the ideal sequence for getting started with this system. It's been tested and proven. It works.

Plan your life and live your plan. LIVE-IT! 180°.

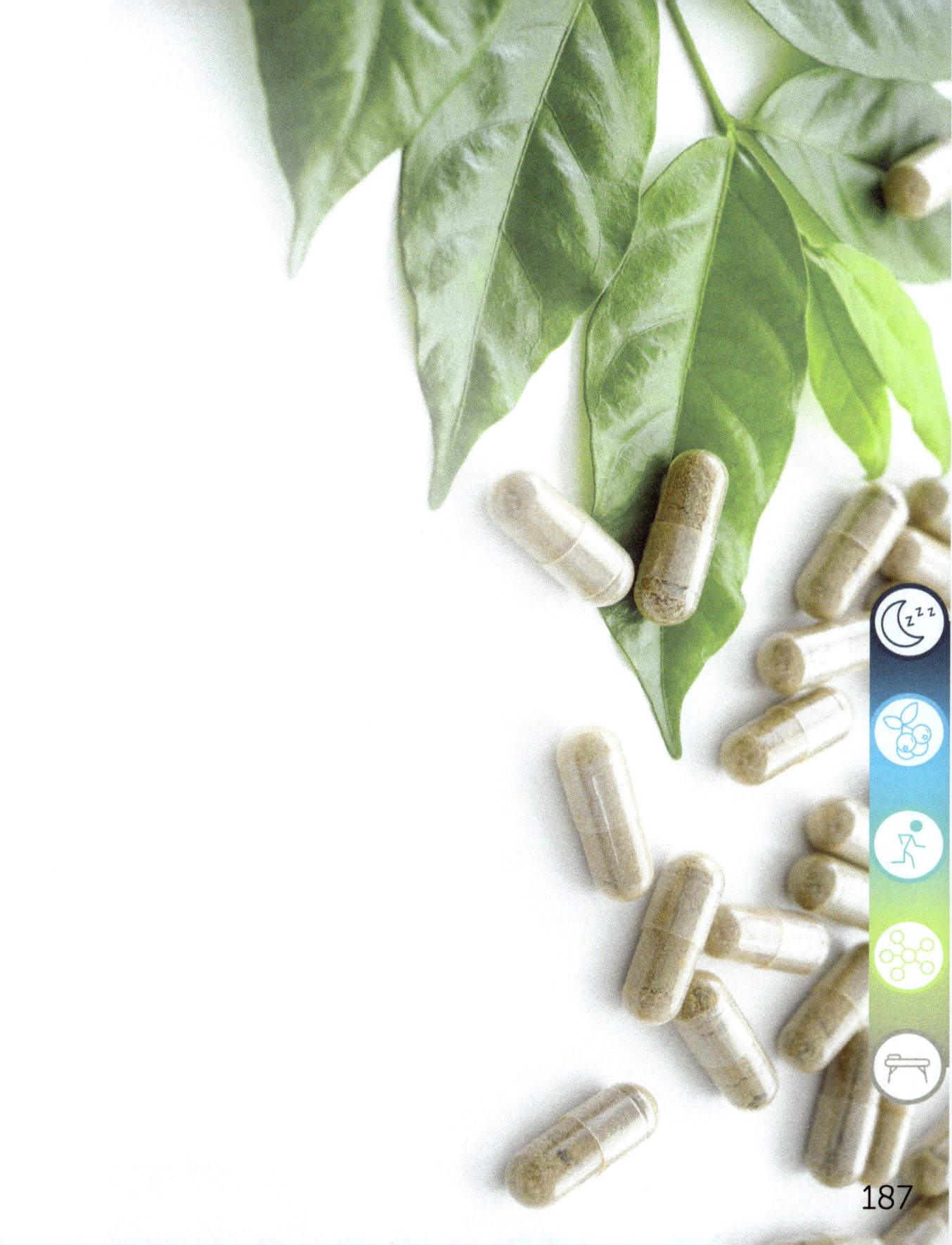

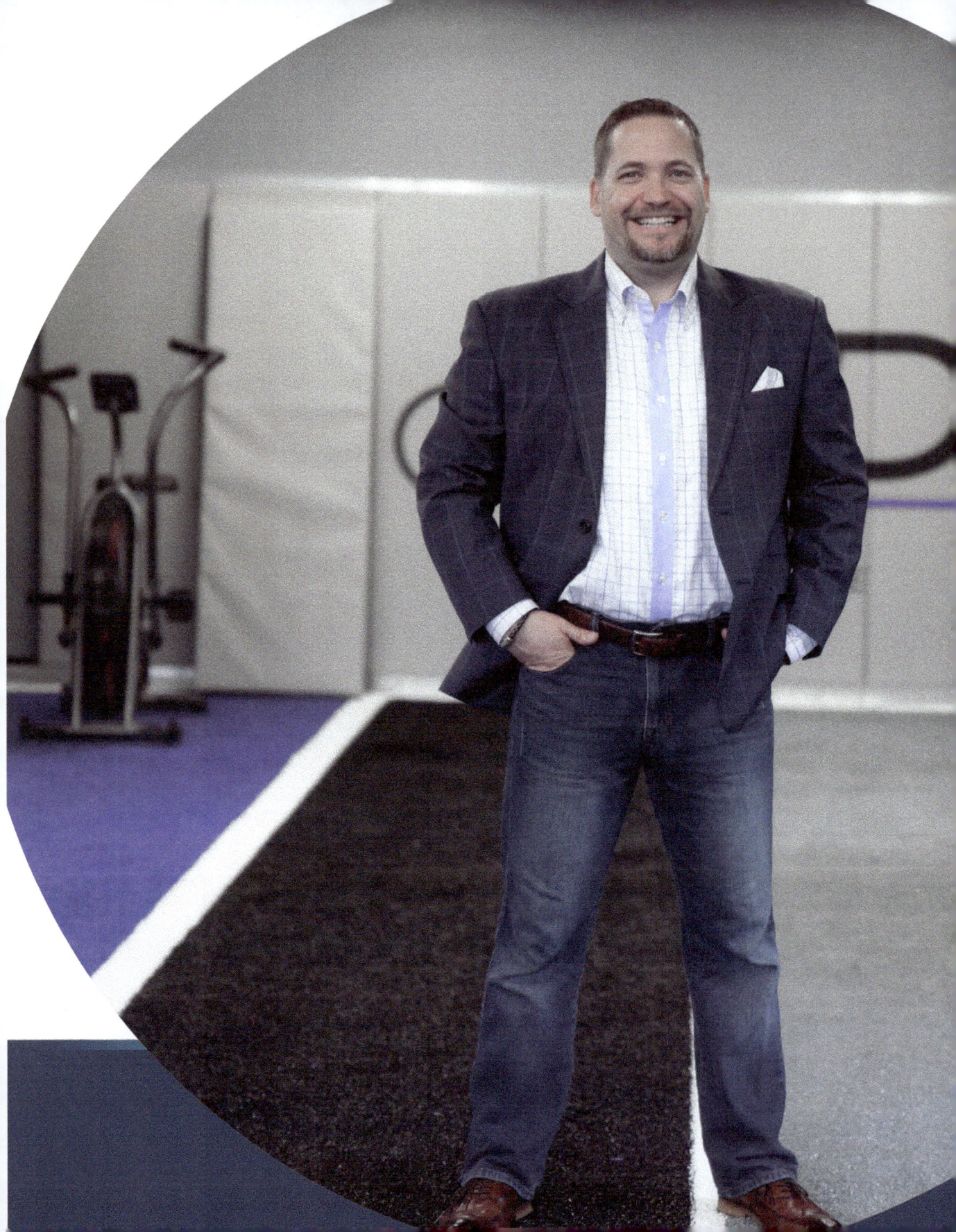

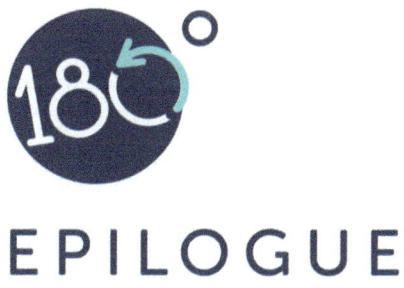

EPILOGUE

I want to remind you of the lesson that saved my life and (who knows) may just save yours: *The choices we make today determine our future.* My belief is that you now have everything you need to get the very most out of the miraculous Intelligently Designed vehicle that is your human body. Specifically, you now have the "owner's manual" necessary to effectively:

RECHARGE
Plug in your body's battery and get back to 100% (by getting enough sleep).

FUEL
Fill your body with quality food (by eating right).

DRIVE
Move your body regularly (by actively using it).

CONNECT
Set your personal destination (by building a sense of purpose and social interaction into your daily life).

REPAIR
Remove the adverse effects of life on your body (by managing stress effectively).

So now you know you've got the perfect car... and you also know you've got the owner's manual you need to get the most you possibly can from that car. What else do you need?

Well, a little perspective about the road ahead is always a good idea.

Let's get real. The road conditions you face in your Intelligently Designed vehicle aren't always going to be ideal. Yes, there are going to be some sunny, beautiful days for driving, some days when you just can't wait to get behind the wheel. But you know what? There are also going to be days when you face blizzards, snow drifts and whiteouts. There are going to be days when heavy rains bring visibility down to almost zero and cause floods that wash out the roads. There are going to be days when you encounter potholes, detours, hail, black ice, massive traffic jams, and any number of other unforeseen difficulties.

In short, there are going to be days when you really don't feel like driving at all. That's reality.

By now, I hope you understand that this feeling is completely normal. The big question is not whether you're going to have days like that, because you are. The big question is how you're going to respond to such days when they happen.

The fact that you had a bad day on the road doesn't mean you put the car keys away and never pick them up again. All that day means is that you had a rough commute. Nothing more. Nothing less. Whenever a day like that comes along, you already know what to do. You acknowledge that tough day for what it is. You cut yourself a little slack. You take the time you need to regroup. And then you get right back out on the road the next morning.

That's the way it works with the car you drive home from work every night. And that's the way it works with the Intelligently Designed vehicle I have been coaching you about in this book. You get back out on the road!

Even people who have successfully made the five critical habits I've shared with you part of their daily lifestyle occasionally have days when they fall off the wagon. That is part of the process. It's part of being human. Every once in a while, we run into a setback, an unexpected obstacle, a series of problems we didn't see coming. WHAM! We look around and realize we have fallen off the wagon. It happens. And when it does, we know exactly what to do. We get right back up on the wagon just as soon as we can. We get back on track. And you can too.

Once you reach the end of this book, you haven't really reached the end of **LIVE-IT! 180°**. You've only reached the beginning. This is the part where you implement what you know, where you accept that you're going to have good days and bad days, where you make this a lifestyle rather than a passing phase. This is the true beginning of this program. It's been my privilege to be your coach up to this point. I hope you will let me continue to support you on the next phase of your journey… because that's where the magic happens.

Please remember that this book, this program, this new way of life is all about choices. Here's the main thing I hope you will take away from everything you've encountered here: I am personally commit-ted to helping you to make the *right* choices in your life… so you can build on the momentum you've already established, dramatically improve the quality of your life, and make the five principles you've learned about in this book part of who you are as a person. It's been an honor and a privilege to be your coach (in book form), and I'm truly proud of you for having made it this far. My next challenge for you is a simple one: Keep our relationship going!

Please visit us at www.liveit180.com and share what you've learned, what you've accomplished, and what has surprised you about this new way of life. You can also email me at coachpete@liveit180.com. Then… let us take this coaching relationship to the next level, with the **LIVE-IT! 180° app** – which you can learn about on the web site or at the iTunes Store or the Google Play Store.

Whatever you choose to do next, my prayer for you is that you continue to make good choices… that you take effective *action* on those choices… and that you become the person you were designed to be.

Lose weight, live fit, enjoy life, and most important, *stay the course*.

> *An idea not coupled with action will never get any bigger than the brain cell it occupied.*
>
> —Arnold Glasow

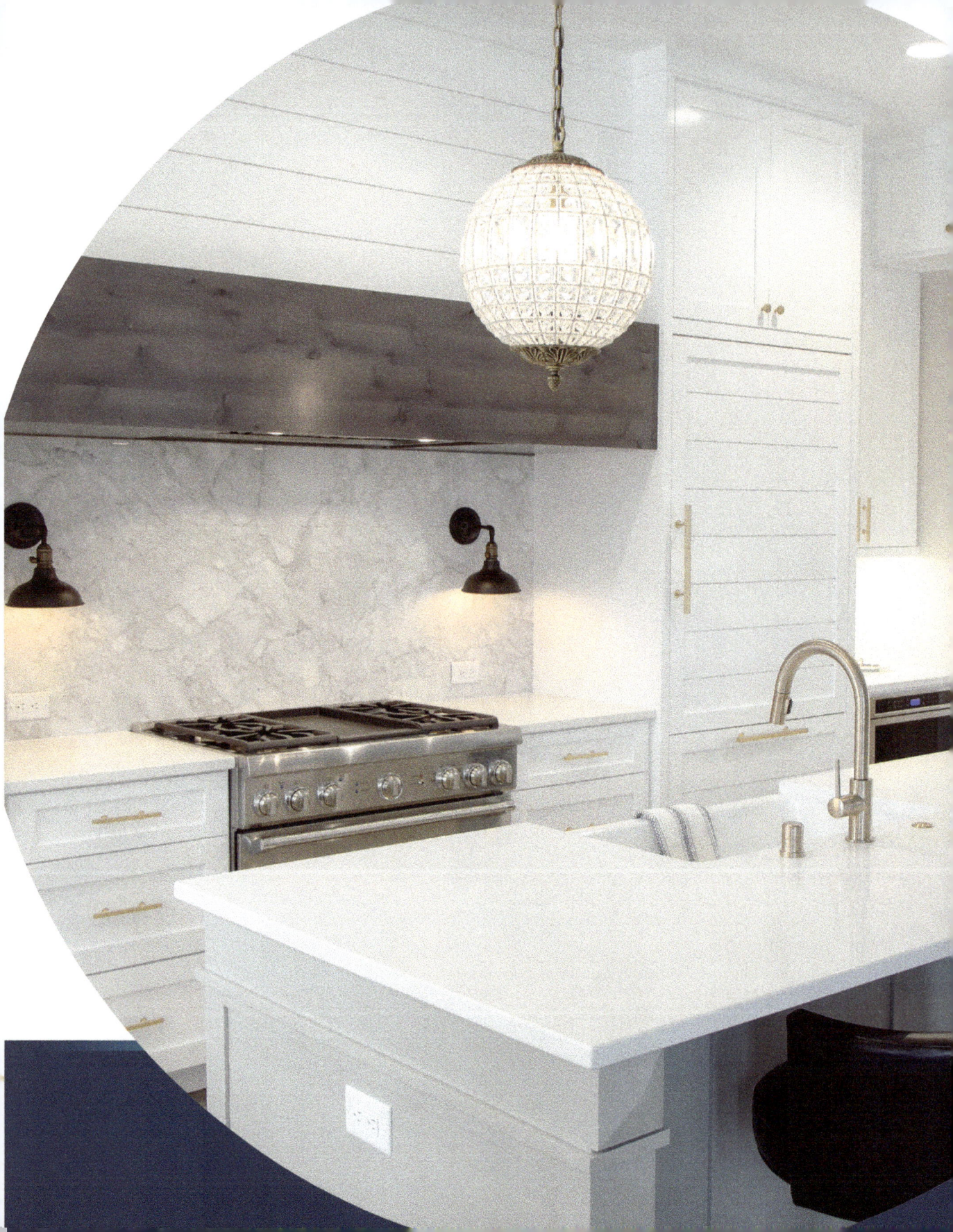

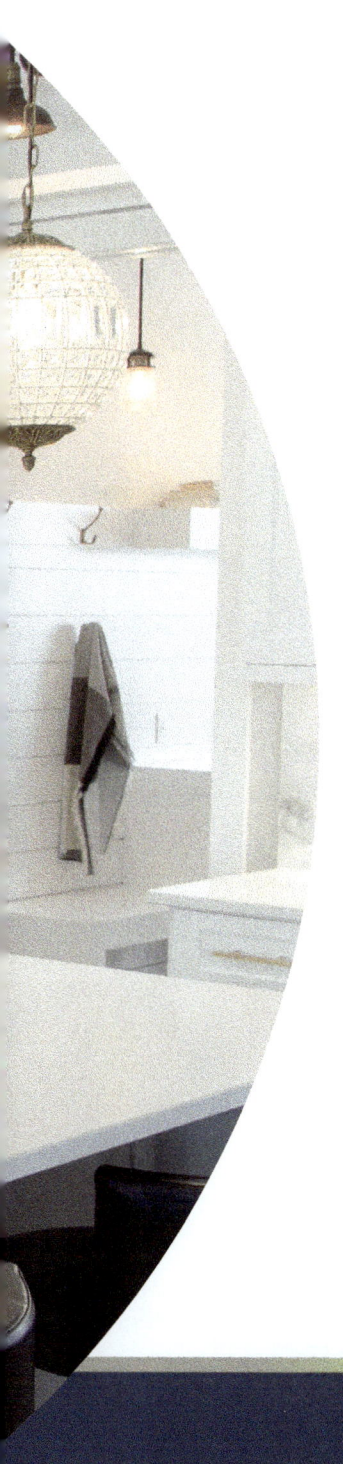

APPENDIX

CLOSE-UP ON YOUR KITCHEN MAKEOVER

Many people ask me, "Why does my kitchen need a makeover? Why can't I do **LIVE-IT! 180°** with the kitchen I already have?"

It's a fair question. The best way to answer it, in my experience, is to pose another question, one that's equally fair – at least in my view. Here it is: If, God forbid, your life went dramatically south, and you found yourself in rehab, trying to shake a major drug habit ... and if, two months later, you managed to make it out of rehab in one piece, clean and sober ... would your chances of *staying* clean and sober go up if you chose to spend *all* your time in places that you knew to be drug-free?

Of course they would. Your odds of cutting that addiction loose for the rest of your life would obviously go up dramatically if you chose to maintain a rigorously drug-free environment. If you were serious about recovery, you would *want* an environment where you didn't run into the bad stuff that had turned your life upside down.

Now, here's a different question, just as relevant: What if you were to make the opposite choice?

Suppose you got out of rehab ... and then, the very next day, you decided that you were going

to spend all your available leisure time hanging around at clubs and parties where there were heavy users of the same stuff that had gotten you into trouble? Would your odds of staying clean and sober go up ... or down?

The answer here is just as obvious. Your chances of living a healthy lifestyle would go

DOWN dramatically if you chose to spend your time hanging out in places where there were lots of illegal, dangerous drugs.

This brings us back to a point I have made repeatedly in this book. Your success or failure with **LIVE-IT! 180°** – as with everything else in life – is all about your choices. And the *choices* you make about your surroundings rank high on the list of importance.

Some people instantly get what I'm talking about when I raise these issues. Others, though, look at me like I'm just a little bit nuts. They ask, "Are you seriously comparing the food that's in my refrigerator and my pantry to the drugs people have to kick when they go into rehab?"

My answer to *that* question is, "Yes. I am." Because guess what? The same basic principle is at work in both situations. Think about it. If you keep doing dangerous, illegal drugs ... what happens to you? You die before your time. If you keep eating all the stuff Big Food makes it easy for you to buy in the average supermarket, in the quantities that Big Food wants you to eat, so that Big Food can keep up its profit margins ... what's going to happen? *You're most likely going to die before your time.*

It's the same outcome! The only real question is how fast it's going to happen.

Here's the bottom line: When you surround yourself with what Big Food tells you to eat, you're throwing the dice with your lifespan and your quality of life, just like a heavy drug user does. Until those dice get done rattling and tumbling and falling, you won't know how quickly the damage you're doing to your body will catch up with you. Why in the world would you choose to accept a risk like that ... by surrounding yourself with bad stuff?

So *yes*, you need to change what's in your pantry, and *yes*, you need to change what's in your refrigerator. Because this is literally a matter of life and death.

As you may remember, LIVE-IT! 180° gives you two weeks to begin the process of making this major change. In this part of the book, I'll provide details on how to implement that change in your kitchen and some practical advice on making it work.

SAD!

The standard American kitchen – which I'm going to assume, from this point forward, is *your* kitchen – supports, by definition, the standard American diet.

Now, the standard American diet is the path of least resistance for most US consumers. Countless nutritionists, physicians, and dietitians refer to this particular way of eating by its acronym: SAD. That's no accident. These experts want that abbreviation to capture your attention.

Because that menu, the menu of least resistance that so many of us follow, really is SAD!

The SAD diet, also known as the "Western pattern" diet, is built on high intakes of red and processed meat, fried foods, high-fat dairy products, refined grains, potatoes, processed foods, and high-sugar or high-fructose corn-syrup drinks. (Any of that in your kitchen? Thought so.)

Studies have shown that this way of eating is correlated, over time, with elevated incidences of obesity, death from heart disease, cancer, (especially colon cancer), Type II diabetes, autoimmune disease, osteoporosis, hypertension, coronary artery disease, and a wide range of inflammatory diseases.

Make no mistake. Dying early and experiencing a severely reduced quality of life during the years before death is what this "diet" can and does lead to for millions of Americans. And that is sad.

In fact, the way most Americans eat is not just sad. It's pathetic. We consume way too many unhealthy fats like trans fats and hydrogenated fats, we ingest a ton of processed foods, we don't get enough fiber, we overload on processed sugars, dairy, and massively refined grains, and we don't eat anywhere near enough vegetables, fruits, or healthy fats.

I hate to be the one to break it to you, but unless you're way ahead of the bell curve, *your kitchen is, right now, perfectly aligned with the SAD diet.*

CLOSE-UP ON YOUR KITCHEN MAKEOVER

Every time you walk into your kitchen, it is practically begging you to consume things like cereal, pastas, and breakfast toaster pastries. It's singing you a siren song about how wonderful dairy products are. It is pointing you toward nitrite- and nitrate-laden meats like hot dogs and salami, and any number of other meats that may look a little less processed but are still loaded with chemicals, antibodies, hormones, and metals (yes, metals). It's inviting you to consume meats that have been genetically modified (GMO) or have been deep-fried within an inch of oblivion. Your kitchen is calling to you, every minute of every hour of every day, to eat all kinds of heavily processed food items of the kind you'll find in the center aisles of the grocery store.

In short, your kitchen is trying to talk you into eating ghost food.

Your kitchen is trying to begin that conversation with you 24 hours a day, 7 days a week. If you are serious about **LIVE-IT! 180°**, which I assume you are, you will need to make your kitchen speak a whole different language.

"HEY, WHERE ARE THE RECIPES?"

Lots of "diet plans" ask you to focus a huge proportion of your energy and attention on studying and following certain recipes. The people who created these plans seem to think cooking the right recipe is the answer to every "dieting" challenge … and they also seem to think that leaving the Standard American Kitchen just as it is presents no real problem.

Although I have plenty of recipes I would love to share with you (and you can ask me about this by emailing coachpete@liveit180.com), I think it's far, far more important to change the *environment* where you prepare your food. If you've got the wrong stuff in the kitchen, you're not going to eat in a healthy way. If you've got the *right* stuff in your kitchen, and if you follow the portion guidelines I've already given you in Chapter Six, you'll be fine.

I believe that, as your coach, it's not my job to make you follow my cookbook or cook my favorite recipes. It is my job, though, to motivate you to transform that kitchen of yours. The very best way I can do that is to let you know, plainly, simply, and in no uncertain terms, that the ghost food you have been trained, over the years, to fill your kitchen with is *just not good for you.*

BRAINWASHED

Unfortunately, we have all been brainwashed into thinking that these foods *are* good for us. Remember the "four basic food groups" so many of us learned about in school? The ones that emphasized grain and dairy consumption? Who do you think was behind that?

Big Food!

In fact, we have been brainwashed so thoroughly that most of us are perfectly okay paying for our lack of education on this issue with a *severely reduced lifespan* ... just so we can avoid challenging or changing something that's become familiar to us.

I realize that the way we typically stock our kitchens is familiar and acceptable to us as a society., and that most people handle the job of stocking the kitchen by buying what is heavily promoted in the supermarket. But you know what? Smoking tobacco in every imaginable public place used to be familiar and acceptable to us as a society too. Just about everyone used to do it. Why? Because Big Tobacco liked it that way. That's why! Eventually, our level of education rose to a point where we realized that the pattern had to change. And that's what needs to happen in our kitchens now. The patterns have to change.

So if you are tempted to push back on what I am saying ... if you are tempted to keep buying what is heavily promoted in the supermarket ... if you are tempted to believe whatever Big Food has paid large sums of money to get you to believe about how good its products are ... if you are tempted to tell me that you can't afford to make the changes I'm about to outline ... I can only say this: **Big Food has been lying to you for decades, and it will continue to lie to you for as long as you will listen.**

I promise you. You *can* afford this. What you can't afford is the status quo.

Big Food is hoping to keep on convincing you to spend your money on junk. And *all* the ghost food in your kitchen is junk. The fact that you are familiar with the process of buying and eating junk is not enough to justify putting your health and well-being at risk.

We have to get off the hamster wheel. We have to make better choices. These foods not only make us sick, foggy brained, exhausted, grouchy, overweight, gassy, bloated, and stricken with headaches and any number of other aches and pains – they also set us up for major diseases that will decimate our quality of life and reduce the number of years we get to spend with our loved ones.

That's what ghost food does, and if you're surrounding yourself with it by putting it in your kitchen, then you need to change your surroundings. That's non-negotiable!

In Chapter Six, you saw three tracks – GOOD, BETTER, and BEST – that pointed you toward healthier food choices. This Appendix is where the rubber meets the road. You're going to put your personalized eating plan into action by committing to one of those tracks ... and you're going to start this journey toward your own personal transformation by transforming your kitchen.

Let me emphasize this point by returning to the rehab analogy. What you experience every day matters. Basically, you're in rehab now. It's not enough for you to be committed to moving in the right direction. In order for you to make

LIVE-IT! 180° INSIGHT

Whether or not you consider the ghost food that's in your kitchen "comfortable," whether or not you feel it's part of your family traditions, whether or not you continue to see it advertised heavily, it has to come out of your kitchen. Why? Because *it is not good for you*. Period.

Shake the Etch-A-Sketch and set up a new design!

LIVE-IT! 180° work, *you have to change the environment*. That means you have to make sure your refrigerator and your pantry are fully committed and on the right track. (And yes, you have to make sure your accountability partner's kitchen is on the right track too.)

Here's how that's going to work.

"GOOD" – PHASE ONE

Your Refrigerator

Relax. Your Kitchen Makeover starts with an instruction that's going to be very, very easy for you to follow. **I want you to give yourself two weeks to eat all the ghost food that's already in your refrigerator.** Enjoy it! Just know you're saying goodbye to it and, following the guidelines below, don't buy any more of it ... unless it falls into one of the three "Easy Exemption" categories you'll be reading about a little later. (Note that these three exemptions are *only* for the GOOD phase of **LIVE-IT! 180°**'s FUEL principle. They're here to make it easy for you to get on track and stay on track.)

Starting immediately, DO NOT restock your refrigerator with any more of the following items:

<u>Prepared Frozen Meals</u>

Begin the process of weaning yourself off Big Food's dubious menu plan by preparing your own meals from scratch. That means no more frozen lasagna, meat loaf, or mac and cheese – in fact, no more frozen prepared meals of any kind. Use up what you have in this heavily processed category, then don't replace any of it. I realize this may be a major lifestyle change. That's good. Make it! Use this two-week period to begin following the healthy "hand portion" eating guidelines I shared with you in Chapter Six.

Soda and Soft Drinks

Heavy consumption of high-calorie drinks is one of the biggest contributors to the climbing obesity rates we see in the western world. So just say no to this stuff! Use the two-week transition period to consume whatever you have on hand, but don't put any more of it in your fridge. And by the way, if you think that bottle of cranberry juice cocktail in your fridge is healthy, think again. After water, its second most prominent ingredient is sugar! And although some people don't want to hear about it, most fruit juices are just as high in sugar as any carbonated soda is. As you'll recall, you've got a lot of water to drink every day as part of **LIVE-IT! 180°**. Make sure you make water your primary beverage. Coffee and green tea are also good.

Nitrite- or Nitrate-laden Meats

The chemicals injected into meats like salami, hot dogs, and processed lunchmeats are very bad news for your body. Don't buy any of them. Use up what you have on hand and don't put any more in your fridge.

Your Pantry

Again, this starts with a guideline that I bet you won't have any trouble at all following: Take two weeks to eat and enjoy all the ghost food that's already in your pantry. Have a blast as you bid all of that stuff farewell. Just don't buy any more of it ... and be sure to check out the three "Easy Exemption" categories I'll be sharing with you in a minute.

(To repeat, these three exemptions are *only* for the GOOD phase of **LIVE-IT! 180°'s** FUEL principle.)

As you begin your two-week transition period, DO NOT restock your pantry with any of the following items:

Cereal that Contain Sugar or High-Fructose Corn Syrup

Your goal in the morning should be to have breakfast – not dessert. Do not replace these items once you use them up.

Prepared Meals (or Pseudo-Meals) that don't Require Refrigeration

This is the corollary of the no-frozen-meals guideline we talked about for your fridge. You're going to choose *not* to replace packages of macaroni and cheese, ramen soup, cup noodles, boxed dinners, and anything else that comes in a package. Instead, you're going to make your meals from scratch.

Cookies, Crackers, Chips and all Other Prepackaged Snack Foods

These heavily processed products are designed to addict you into consuming them in large quantities. Have some chopped carrots with hummus instead.

Peanut Butter

Even the organic kind that's composed of 100% peanuts. Why? Because, as I noted earlier, the peanuts used in peanut butter sometimes have serious quality and inspection problems ... and because there has been research that links some cancers with peanut butter. Coincidence? Maybe not!

For suggestions on what you should buy and eat instead of the foods listed above, during the GOOD phase Consult the grocery list you'll find at the end of this Appendix. And don't just read about it. *Execute* this plan. Be sure your accountability partner supports you fully as you take action to make these major changes in your lifestyle ... and that you support him or her in the same way!

The Three Easy Exemptions

Here is the lowdown on the three Easy Exemptions you can give yourself in the GOOD phase.

Easy Exemption #1: Dairy

Q. Can I replace dairy items (milk, cheese, yogurt and so on) that I use up?

A. While you are implementing the GOOD phase of the FUEL principle, the answer to this is yes, *if*...

» You notice how much dairy you consumed during your two-week transition period ... and reduce your dairy consumption in comparison. How much you reduce it by is up to you.

» You don't buy or consume ice cream or frozen yogurt products. These products contain too much sugar and/or high-fructose corn syrup and too many weird additives.

» You keep your accountability partner up-do-date with the specific choices you've made about your dairy consumption and get his or her feedback.

Easy Exemption #2: Sugar

Q. Can I replace items that are high in sugar and/or high-fructose corn syrup that I use up?

A. While you are implementing the GOOD phase of the EAT principle, the answer to this is yes, *if*...

» You notice how much sugar and high-fructose corn syrup you consumed during the two-week transition period ... and reduce your consumption of these products. Again, how much you reduce them by is up to you. Just make sure the amount consumed each week goes down. (Yes, this means you need to get used to checking labels carefully.)

» You continue to avoid sodas, soft drinks, and fruit juice, instead drinking water at the levels I recommended. This one lifestyle change will have an immediate positive impact on your energy level and your overall health and well-being.

» You keep your accountability partner up-do-date with the specific choices you've made about your consumption of products that include sugar and high-fructose corn syrup and ask for his or her feedback.

Easy Exemption #3: Bread, Pasta, and other Grain-Based Products

Q. Can I replace bread, pasta and grain items that I use up?

A. While you are implementing the GOOD phase of the FUEL principle, the answer to this is yes, if...

» You notice how much bread, pasta, and grain-based products you consumed during your two-week transition period ... and reduce your consumption of those items going forward by *half*.

» You keep your accountability partner up-do-date with the choices you've made about your consumption of bread, pasta, and grain items and continue to get his or her feedback.

(A side note: Here in the GOOD phase, you can continue to buy bread items even if they contain ingredients that you don't understand. That's just a nod to convenience.)

At this point, you have the blueprint for a very basic Kitchen Makeover, the kind that will support you fully while you're in the GOOD phase. If you do only this much – and I've gone out of my way to make it relatively easy for you to do – you will be on track to successfully execute all three phases of the EAT principle, because your kitchen and your accountability partner will support you.

LIVE-IT! 180° TIP

For further help and support on your Kitchen Makeover, reach out to us at Liveit180.com.

"BETTER" – PHASE TWO

Your Refrigerator

Once you move on to the next phase of the FUEL principle, you will build on all the work you did back in the GOOD phase … and you'll make sure the contents of your refrigerator support you as you do. That means you'll be eliminating…

<u>Processed Foods You are Supposed to Freeze or Chill</u>

This means *anything* that comes in a box, carton, or wrapper and is meant to go into your refrigerator. Here at the BETTER phase, you will start saying no to *all* this packaged stuff. Do not put it on the grocery list. Do not buy it. Do not bring it into your house. I realize this is probably one of the biggest pattern interrupts you'll be making, because most of us have grown up believing that buying and eating processed food is how we're supposed to live. Actually, it's *not!* Processed food is typically three to seven steps away from the good earth, and it's typically loaded with all kinds of weird ingredients, some of which hardly anybody can pronounce! You want food that's only one to two steps away from the good earth, food that nobody has decided to lace with strange substances in order to cut processing costs or get you addicted to the product in question. This means staying away from *all* frozen dinners, frozen breakfasts, frozen desserts, frozen entrees, frozen appetizers, and frozen bags of fruits and vegetables. (Buy fresh fruits and vegetables instead!)

The frozen food aisle is where Big Food sneaks in a lot of its strange additions to the national food supply. Case in point: One of my clients found a pre-packaged frozen meat offering containing 15 grams of protein *and* 15 grams of carbohydrate per serving. I was curious. Where the heck was all that carbohydrate coming from? When I inspected the label, I found that sugar had been added to every single meatball. Why was it there? To get people hooked on sweet meatballs and keep them coming back for more. Needless to say, we sent that package back. Still more insidious are the ubiquitous "artificial colors and flavors" your government is perfectly okay with Big Food pumping into its products, even if that means that what ends up in your fridge and/or freezer is made from plastic, petroleum, paper pulp, or cow manure. So, stop putting this stuff in your refrigerator and stop eating it.

<u>Fruits and Vegetables that are not Fresh</u>

In this phase, you're going to begin a pattern of eating *only* fresh fruits and vegetables (nothing canned or frozen). The goal here is, for *most* of the fruits and vegetables you consume, to start buying produce that is explicitly labeled "organic." That means no synthetic pesticides, chemical fertilizers, or genetic modification. You may be able to get good organic options for your fruits and vegetables at your local supermarket. If not, head to your local farmer's market. Be sure to buy all your fruits and vegetables *in season*, no matter where you shop.

Dairy

Milk and milk products are no longer part of your eating routine here in the BETTER phase. Try the almond milk! Eggs are okay, just be sure to follow the protein quantity guidelines I laid out for you in Chapter Six.

Your Pantry

Here in the BETTER phase, your pantry will declare itself "off-limits" to the following:

Processed Foods that Come in a Box, Carton, or Wrapper

Same deal here as with your fridge. These products are Big Food's favorite places to hide strange ingredients that aren't good for you, so you're going to stop buying them. That means that, in addition to the cereals, ready-made meals, and snacks that you declared off-limits in the GOOD phase, you'll be buying no more packages of Pop Tarts, dried mashed potatoes, microwave popcorn, or anything else with an indecipherable ingredient list. This stuff is usually found in the middle aisles of the grocery store. If it comes in a box, carton, or wrapper and it has a long list of ingredients that includes items you can't pronounce or artificial colors or artificial flavors, you're not going to buy it anymore. End of story.

Canned Fruits and Vegetables

Yes, you can use up what you have on hand. Just replace it with the fresh stuff. Remember that, in **LIVE-IT! 180°**, you get to eat as many vegetables as you want. Once you gobble up all your canned goods, feel free to chow down on those chopped carrots!

Processed Grains and Bread Made from Wheat or Wheat Flour

Here at the BETTER phase, you're going to limit your grain consumption to corn and brown rice, and if you want, bread or pastry made from coconut flour, almond flour, or cashew flour. See Chapter Six for details.

Important

You will also severely limit purchases of sugar and other sweeteners at this stage, reducing your consumption of these to something between 45 and 60 grams per day. Assume that your fruit consumption will contribute 15 grams. Note that a single teaspoon of sugar is 4.2 grams of sugar! So, if you put two teaspoons of sugar in your coffee, be aware that you're already up to about 8 grams.

Speaking of coffee, you don't need to eliminate it from your grocery list at the BETTER phase, but you will want to cut back on it. Your aim is to consume *half* as much caffeine per day as you did during the GOOD phase.

Talk with your accountability partner regularly about all the changes you are making in your kitchen.

"BEST" – PHASE THREE

Your Refrigerator

Once you move into the final phase of the FUEL principle, you will take your lifestyle to a whole new level. Make sure your refrigerator supports your choices. Follow all the BETTER guidelines, and transition away from…

Meat and Poultry that Contains Additives or Hormones or has been Genetically Modified

At this level, you're going to shift to buying *only* organic produce and meat. In other words, you are choosing *not* to put synthetic pesticides, chemical fertilizers, hormones, antibiotics, and GMOs into your system. So, keep that stuff out of your fridge.

Regular-Layer Eggs

Here at the BEST phase, you will switch to Omega-3 eggs, laid by chickens fed an Omega-3 rich diet. These eggs are enriched with essential polyunsaturated fats. Alternatively, you can head down to the local farmer's market or nearby farm and purchase eggs laid by chickens that are allowed to roam and graze. The best of both worlds would be free-range eggs rich in Omega-3 nutrients, which some stores now carry.

Your Pantry

Here at the BEST phase, you'll need to make a couple more changes to your larder. In addition to the changes you made in the BETTER phase, you should now only purchase products with no more than *five* ingredients, all of them pronounceable. You will also want to eliminate the following:

All Grain

Yes, you can do it. Your large intestine with thank you! See Chapter Six for details on this. For some innovative ideas that will help you to wean yourself off grain, you can email me at coachpete@liveit180.com.

Most Caffeine

The maximum intake is one cup of coffee a day.

Most Sugar and High-Fructose Corn Syrup

The maximum intake of this is 45 grams a day.

MAKE IT HAPPEN!

Here's my promise to you: If you make the effort to transform your kitchen environment as I've outlined, and if you keep in touch with your accountability partner every step of the way, you will unlock a daily lifestyle that gives you more vibrant energy, more optimism, more *possibility* than you ever dreamed possible … because what I've outlined here is based on the way your body is Intelligently Designed to operate! Try it for yourself and see.

PUTTING TOGETHER YOUR WEEKLY GROCERY LIST

The following is a list of items you could include on a weekly grocery list suitable for a family of one to two adults. These items have been tested extensively with good results. Adapt the list to the phase you are in — GOOD, BETTER, or BEST — and to your own world, by making appropriate, responsible additions. Some of the items on the list may seem unusual to you. Nonetheless, I ask you to consider them. You don't have to follow this list to the letter, but I recommend that you take a good, long look at it *before* you begin shopping for the GOOD phase. Use it to get clearer in your own mind about the direction in which you — and your kitchen — are headed.

As you shop, take note of the path of travel through the store. You'll likely notice that the healthiest items are located on the *periphery* of the store … and that the ones I have urged you to get rid of tend to be located near the center. Here's my advice: Make life easy on yourself. Stick to the outer regions of the supermarket!

ITEMS YOU COULD INCLUDE ON YOUR GROCERY LIST

Oil (Organic if Possible)

- ☐ Avocado
- ☐ Coconut
- ☐ Olive

Vegetables (Organic if Possible)

- ☐ Artichoke
- ☐ Arugula
- ☐ Asparagus
- ☐ Avocado
- ☐ Beets
- ☐ Bok Choy
- ☐ Broccoli (All Forms)
- ☐ Brussel Sprouts
- ☐ Cabbage
- ☐ Carrots
- ☐ Cauliflower
- ☐ Celery
- ☐ Collards
- ☐ Cucumbers
- ☐ Eggplant
- ☐ Endives
- ☐ Fennel
- ☐ Garlic
- ☐ Green Beans
- ☐ Jicama
- ☐ Kale
- ☐ Kohlrabi
- ☐ Leeks
- ☐ Mushrooms
- ☐ Mustard Greens
- ☐ Onions
- ☐ Parsnip
- ☐ Peppers (All Forms)
- ☐ Pumpkin
- ☐ Radish
- ☐ Lettuce (All Forms)
- ☐ Rutabaga
- ☐ Sea Vegetables
- ☐ Spinach
- ☐ Squash
- ☐ Sweet Potatoes
- ☐ Swiss Chard
- ☐ Tomatoes
- ☐ Turnip Greens
- ☐ Watercress
- ☐ Yams
- ☐ Zucchini

Protein

Fish (Wild – NO Farm Raised)

- ☐ Anchovies
- ☐ Bass
- ☐ Cod
- ☐ Eel
- ☐ Haddock
- ☐ Halibut
- ☐ Herring
- ☐ Mackerel
- ☐ Mahi Mahi
- ☐ Monkfish

- [ ] Mullet
- [ ] Northern Pike
- [ ] Perch
- [ ] Red Snapper
- [ ] Rock Fish
- [ ] Salmon
- [ ] Sardines
- [ ] Tuna
- [ ] Walleye
- [ ] Wild fish (All Forms)

Meat (Free Range, Organic, Lean)

- [ ] Alligator
- [ ] Bear
- [ ] Beef
- [ ] Bison
- [ ] Caribou
- [ ] Chicken
- [ ] Duck
- [ ] Elk
- [ ] Emu
- [ ] Goat
- [ ] Goose
- [ ] Kangaroo
- [ ] Lamb
- [ ] Ostrich
- [ ] Pheasant
- [ ] Pork
- [ ] Quail
- [ ] Rabbit
- [ ] Turkey
- [ ] Venison

Eggs (Free Range, Organic)

- [ ] Chicken
- [ ] Duck
- [ ] Emu
- [ ] Goose
- [ ] Pheasant
- [ ] Quail

Shellfish (Wild – Not Farm Raised)

- [ ] Abalone
- [ ] Clams
- [ ] Crab
- [ ] Crayfish
- [ ] Lobster
- [ ] Mussels
- [ ] Oysters
- [ ] Prawns
- [ ] Scallops
- [ ] Shrimp

Fruits (Organic if Possible)

- [ ] Acai
- [ ] Apples
- [ ] Ackees
- [ ] Apricots
- [ ] Bananas
- [ ] Bilberries
- [ ] Blackberries
- [ ] Blackcurrants
- [ ] Blueberries

- [ ] Boysenberries
- [ ] Currants
- [ ] Cherries
- [ ] Cranberries
- [ ] Dates
- [ ] Dragon Fruits
- [ ] Elderberries
- [ ] Figs
- [ ] Goji Berries
- [ ] Gooseberries
- [ ] Grapes
- [ ] Honey Berries
- [ ] Huckleberries
- [ ] Jackfruits
- [ ] Juniper Berries
- [ ] Kiwifruits
- [ ] Kumquats
- [ ] Lemons
- [ ] Limes
- [ ] Lychees
- [ ] Mangos
- [ ] Melons (All Forms)
- [ ] Mulberries
- [ ] Nectarines
- [ ] Oranges (All Forms)
- [ ] Papayas
- [ ] Passionfruit
- [ ] Peaches
- [ ] Pears
- [ ] Plantains
- [ ] Plums
- [ ] Pineapples
- [ ] Pomegranates
- [ ] Quinces
- [ ] Raspberries
- [ ] Redcurrants
- [ ] Soursops
- [ ] Star Apples
- [ ] Star Fruits
- [ ] Strawberries
- [ ] Tamarinds

Good Fats (Organic if Possible)

- [ ] Avocados
- [ ] Chia Seeds
- [ ] Coconuts (All Forms – Including Oil)
- [ ] Dark Chocolates (No Sugar)
- [ ] Flaxseeds
- [ ] Nuts (All Forms – No Peanuts)
- [ ] Nut Butters (All Forms – No Peanuts)
- [ ] Olives (All Forms – Including Oil)
- [ ] Seeds (All Forms)

Non-Dairy Milk (Organic if Possible)

- [ ] Almond
- [ ] Cashew
- [ ] Coconut
- [ ] Macadamia

Spices/Herbs:

No restrictions - all are good

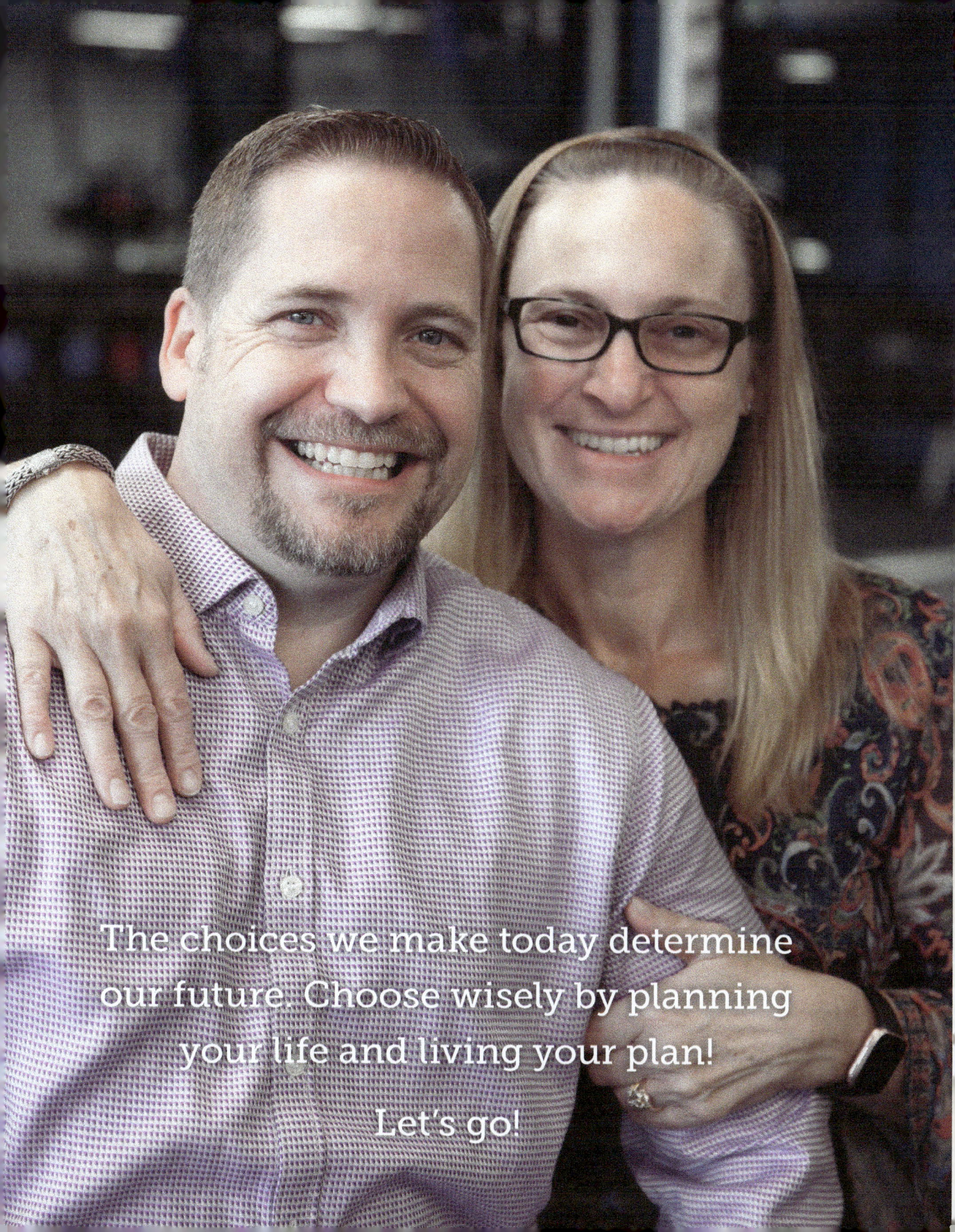

www.ingramcontent.com/pod-product-compliance
Lightning Source LLC
Chambersburg PA
CBHW051616030426
42334CB00030B/3221